National Certified Phlebotomy Technician Exam

SECRETS

Study Guide

Your Key to Exam Success

NCCT Test Review for the
National Center for Competency
Testing Exam

Dear Future Exam Success Story:

Congratulations on your purchase of our study guide. Our goal in writing our study guide was to cover the content on the test, as well as provide insight into typical test taking mistakes and how to overcome them.

Standardized tests are a key component of being successful, which only increases the importance of doing well in the high-pressure high-stakes environment of test day. How well you do on this test will have a significant impact on your future, and we have the research and practical advice to help you execute on test day.

The product you're reading now is designed to exploit weaknesses in the test itself, and help you avoid the most common errors test takers frequently make.

How to use this study guide

We don't want to waste your time. Our study guide is fast-paced and fluff-free. We suggest going through it a number of times, as repetition is an important part of learning new information and concepts.

First, read through the study guide completely to get a feel for the content and organization. Read the general success strategies first, and then proceed to the content sections. Each tip has been carefully selected for its effectiveness.

Second, read through the study guide again, and take notes in the margins and highlight those sections where you may have a particular weakness.

Finally, bring the manual with you on test day and study it before the exam begins.

Your success is our success

We would be delighted to hear about your success. Send us an email and tell us your story. Thanks for your business and we wish you continued success.

Sincerely,

Mometrix Test Preparation Team

Need more help? Check out our flashcards at: http://MometrixFlashcards.com/NCCT

TABLE OF CONTENTS

Top 20 Test Taking Tips

1. Carefully follow all the test registration procedures
2. Know the test directions, duration, topics, question types, how many questions
3. Setup a flexible study schedule at least 3-4 weeks before test day
4. Study during the time of day you are most alert, relaxed, and stress free
5. Maximize your learning style; visual learner use visual study aids, auditory learner use auditory study aids
6. Focus on your weakest knowledge base
7. Find a study partner to review with and help clarify questions
8. Practice, practice, practice
9. Get a good night's sleep; don't try to cram the night before the test
10. Eat a well balanced meal
11. Know the exact physical location of the testing site; drive the route to the site prior to test day
12. Bring a set of ear plugs; the testing center could be noisy
13. Wear comfortable, loose fitting, layered clothing to the testing center; prepare for it to be either cold or hot during the test
14. Bring at least 2 current forms of ID to the testing center
15. Arrive to the test early; be prepared to wait and be patient
16. Eliminate the obviously wrong answer choices, then guess the first remaining choice
17. Pace yourself; don't rush, but keep working and move on if you get stuck
18. Maintain a positive attitude even if the test is going poorly
19. Keep your first answer unless you are positive it is wrong
20. Check your work, don't make a careless mistake

Anatomy/Physiology

Growth Hormone

Growth Hormone (GH, somatotropin) - controlled by both releasing and inhibiting hormones, GHRH and GHIH (somatostatin), from the hypothalamus. GH causes growth and development of the musculoskeletal system and other tissues. It stimulates amino acids to be used for protein synthesis and causes lipolysis to provide fatty acids for catabolism. For these reasons it is sometimes abused to stimulate muscle growth and catabolize fat. Negative feedback results from GH itself and also from mediators called somatomedins (Somatomedin is also known as Insulin-like Growth Factor produced by the liver, muscles, and other tissue. Positive feedback is produced by strenuous exercise and energy demanding activities.

Childhood hypersecretion of GH causes the excessive growth seen in gigantism, adulthood hypersecretion causes acromegaly, a condition in which the bones are exaggerated in shape. Hyposecretion in childhood causes dwarfism.

Skeletal System

There are about 206 bones in the human body, they function to protect and preserve the shape of soft tissues. The skeleton provides a framework for the muscles, it controls and directs internal pressure and provides stability anchoring points for other soft tissues. There are a wide variety of bones/bony tissues adapted for specific functions to aid locomotion and support; bones are moved by the skeletal muscles. In addition the skeletal system stores and produces blood cells in the bone marrow.

There are two types of bone tissue: compact and spongy. The names imply that the two types of differ in density, or how tightly the tissue is packed together. There are three types of cells that contribute to bone homeostasis. Osteoblasts are bone-forming cell, osteoclasts resorb or break down bone, and osteocytes are mature bone cells. Equilibrium between osteoblasts and osteoclasts maintains bone tissue.

Compact Bone
Compact bone consists of closely packed osteons or haversian systems. The osteon consists of a central canal called the osteonic (haversian) canal, which is surrounded

by concentric rings (lamellae) of matrix. Between the rings of matrix, the bone cells (osteocytes) are located in spaces called lacunae. Small channels (canaliculi) radiate from the lacunae to the osteonic (haversian) canal to provide passageways through the hard matrix. In compact bone, the haversian systems are packed tightly together to form what appears to be a solid mass. The osteonic canals contain blood vessels that are parallel to the long axis of the bone. These blood vessels interconnect, by way of perforating canals, with vessels on the surface of the bone.

Spongy Bone

Spongy (cancellous) bone is lighter and less dense than compact bone. Spongy bone consists of plates (trabeculae) and bars of bone adjacent to small, irregular cavities that contain red bone marrow. The canaliculi connect to the adjacent cavities, instead of a central haversian canal, to receive their blood supply. It may appear that the trabeculae are arranged in a haphazard manner, but they are organized to provide maximum strength similar to braces that are used to support a building. The trabeculae of spongy bone follow the lines of stress and can realign if the direction of stress changes.

Muscular System

The muscular system is composed of specialized cells called muscle fibers. Muscle fibers predominant function is contractibility. Muscles, where attached to bones or internal organs and blood vessels, are responsible for movement. Nearly all movement in the body is the result of muscle contraction.

The muscular system in human consists of three different types of muscles: cardiac, skeletal and smooth.
- Cardiac muscle is a striated muscle that makes up the heart. It is the only type of muscle consisting of branching fibers.
- Skeletal muscle consists of voluntary muscles attached to the frame of the skeletal system enabling bodily movement.
- Smooth muscle is the involuntary muscle that enables the movement of internal organs.

Movement of most muscles is controlled through the nervous system, although some muscles (such as cardiac muscle) can be completely autonomous. There are about 70,000 muscles in the human body

Reproduction System

The major function of the reproductive system is to ensure survival of the species. This is carried out by four following objectives.

- To produce egg and sperm cells
- To transport and sustain these cells
- To nurture the developing offspring
- To produce hormones

Female reproductive terms:

- <u>Uterus</u>- The hollow female reproductive organ in which a fertilized egg is implanted and a fetus develops also know as the womb
- <u>Fallopian Tubes</u>- two thin tubes that extend from each side of the uterus, toward the ovaries, as a passageway for eggs and sperm
- <u>Ova</u>- A female sex cell, or egg
- <u>Cervix</u>- the neck of the womb located at the top of the vagina
- <u>Ovaries</u>- The female sex gland with both a reproductive function (releasing ova) and a hormonal function (production of estrogen and progesterone)

Digestive System

The digestive system includes the digestive tract and its accessory organs, which process food into molecules that can be absorbed and utilized by the cells of the body. Food is broken down, bit by bit, until the molecules are small enough to be absorbed and the waste products are eliminated. The digestive tract, also called the alimentary canal or gastrointestinal (GI) tract, consists of a long continuous tube that extends from the mouth to the anus. It includes the mouth, pharynx, esophagus, stomach, small intestine, and large intestine. The tongue and teeth are accessory structures located in the mouth. The Salivary glands, liver, and gallbladder pancreas are major accessory organs that have a role in digestion. These organs secrete fluids into the digestive tract.

Functions of the Digestive System:

- *Movement* -- After ingestion and mastication, the food particles move from the mouth into the pharynx, then into the esophagus. This movement is deglutition or swallowing. Mixing movements occur in the stomach as a result of smooth muscle contraction. These repetitive contractions usually occur in small segments of the digestive tract and mix the food particles with

-4-

enzymes and other fluids. The movements that propel the food particles through the digestive tract are called peristalsis. These are rhythmic waves of contractions that move the food particles through the various regions in which mechanical and chemical digestion takes place.

- *Absorption* -- The simple molecules that result from chemical digestion pass through cell membranes of the lining in the small intestine into the blood or lymph capillaries. This process is called absorption.
- *Elimination* -- The food molecules that cannot be digested or absorbed need to be eliminated from the body. The removal of indigestible wastes through the anus, in the form of feces, is defecation or elimination.
- *Ingestion* -- The first activity of the digestive system is to take in food through the mouth. This process, called ingestion, has to take place before anything else can happen.
- *Mechanical Digestion* -- The large pieces of food that are ingested have to be broken into smaller particles that can be acted upon by various enzymes. This is mechanical digestion, which begins in the mouth with chewing or mastication and continues with churning and mixing actions in the stomach.
- *Chemical Digestion* -- The complex molecules of carbohydrates, proteins, and fats are transformed by chemical digestion into smaller molecules that can be absorbed and utilized by the cells. Chemical digestion, through a process called hydrolysis, uses water and digestive enzymes to break down the complex molecules. Digestive enzymes speed up the hydrolysis process, which is otherwise very slow.

Endocrine System

The endocrine system functions in the regulation of body activities. The endocrine system acts through chemical messengers called hormones that influence growth, development, and metabolic activities. The action of the endocrine system is measured in minutes, hours, or weeks. The endocrine system works with the nervous system to maintain homeostasis in the body.
There are two major categories of glands in the body - exocrine and endocrine.

- *Exocrine Glands* -- Exocrine glands have ducts that carry their secretory product to a surface. These glands include the sweat, sebaceous, and mammary glands and, the glands that secrete digestive enzymes.

- *Endocrine Glands* -- The endocrine glands do not have ducts to carry their product to a surface. They are called ductless glands. The word endocrine is derived from the Greek terms "endo," meaning within, and "krine," meaning to separate or secrete.

The secretory products of endocrine glands are called hormones and are secreted directly into the blood and then carried throughout the body where they influence only those cells that have receptor sites for that hormone.

Nervous System

The nervous system is the major controlling, regulatory, and communicating system in the body. It is the center of all mental activity including thought, learning, and memory. Together with the endocrine system, the nervous system is responsible for regulating and maintaining homeostasis. Through its receptors, the nervous system keeps us in touch with our environment, both external and internal. The three main functions of the nervous system are sensory, integrative and motor. Sensory part of the nervous system detects changes in the external environment like temperature, light and sound. It also monitors the internal environment such as blood pressure, pH, CO_2 level, and electrolyte levels. The input into the sensory system is called stimuli. Integration occurs when the stimuli from the sensory system is processed by the brain into create memories, thoughts, sensations, and decisions. Motor describes the response of the body due to the integration of the stimuli. This can result in the movement of a muscle or the release of a hormone from a gland.

Peripheral Nervous System
The organs of the peripheral nervous system are the nerves and ganglia. Nerves are bundles of nerve fibers, much like muscles are bundles of muscle fibers. Cranial nerves and spinal nerves extend from the CNS to peripheral organs such as muscles and glands. Ganglia are collections, or small knots, of nerve cell bodies outside the CNS. The peripheral nervous system is further subdivided into an afferent (sensory) division and an efferent (motor) division. The afferent or sensory division transmits impulses from peripheral organs to the CNS. The efferent or motor division transmits impulses from the CNS out to the peripheral organs to cause an effect or action. Finally, the efferent or motor division is again subdivided into the somatic nervous system and the autonomic nervous system. The somatic nervous system, also called the somatomotor or somatic efferent nervous system, supplies motor impulses to the skeletal muscles. Because these nerves permit conscious control of

- 6 -

the skeletal muscles, it is sometimes called the voluntary nervous system. The autonomic nervous system, also called the visceral efferent nervous system, supplies motor impulses to cardiac muscle, to smooth muscle, and to glandular epithelium. It is further subdivided into sympathetic and parasympathetic divisions. Because the autonomic nervous system regulates involuntary or automatic functions, it is called the involuntary nervous system.

Central Nervous System

The brain and spinal cord are the organs of the central nervous system. Because they are so vitally important, the brain and spinal cord, located in the dorsal body cavity, are encased in bone for protection. The brain is in the cranial vault, and the spinal cord is in the vertebral canal of the vertebral column. Although considered to be two separate organs, the brain and spinal cord are continuous at the foramen magnum.

Urinary System

The principal function of the urinary system is to maintain the volume and composition of body fluids within normal limits. One aspect of this function is to rid the body of waste products that accumulate as a result of cellular metabolism and because of this, it is sometimes referred to as the excretory system. The urinary system maintains an appropriate fluid volume by regulating the amount of water that is excreted in the urine. Other aspects of its function include regulating the concentrations of various electrolytes in the body fluids and maintaining normal pH of the blood. In addition to maintaining fluid homeostasis in the body, the urinary system controls red blood cell production by secreting the hormone erythropoietin. The urinary system also plays a role in maintaining normal blood pressure by secreting the enzyme renin.

Integumentary System

The integumentary system contains the largest organ in the human body, the skin. It is also comprised of such extensions of the skin as hair and fingernails. The skin, however, is the most important of these. The skin protects and cushions the body's delicate organs. It also provides the body a physical barrier to keep out foreign materials, to prevent the body from drying out, and to assist with the regulation of body temperature.

Epidermis

The epidermis, as its name suggests, is the outermost layer of the skin. It is comprised of four separate layers of epithelial tissue. The outermost layer of the epidermis is the stratum corneum. It is approximately 20-30 cells thick. The cells here are completely keratinized and dead, and this is what gives the skin its waterproof quality. The next two layers, the stratum granulosum and the stratum lucidum, are similar in that they represent an intermediate stage of keratinization. The cells here are not fully keratinized yet, but as the growth of the skin pushes them outward, they will increasingly move towards that state. The deepest layer of the epidermis is the stratum germinativum. The cells here are mitotically active-- that is, they are alive and reproducing. This is where the growth of skin takes place.

Major structures found in skin:

- Pore -- A tiny opening in the skin that serves as an outlet for sweat
- Sweat gland -- Any of the glands in the skin that secrete perspiration usually located in the dermis
- Nerve ending -- The terminal structure of an axon that does not end at a synapse
- Erector pili -- Tiny smooth muscle fibers attached to each hair follicle, which contract to make the hairs stand on end
- Hair follicle -- A hair follicle is part of the skin that grows hair by packing old cells together. Inside the follicle the sebaceous gland is found. At the end of the hair, tiny blood vessels form the root, around the root there is a white structure called a bulb, which is visible on plucked healthy hairs.
- Sebaceous gland -- A gland in the skin that opens into a hair follicle and secretes an oily substance called sebum

Dermis and subcutaneous layers of skin:

- *Dermis* -- The dermis is the second layer of skin, directly beneath the epidermis. Unlike the epidermis, the dermis has its own blood supply. Sweat glands are present to collect water and various wastes from the bloodstream, and excrete them through pores in the epidermis. The dermis is also the site of hair roots, and it is here where the growth of hair takes place. By the time hair reaches the environment outside of the skin, it has died. The dermis also contains dense connective tissue, made of collagen fibers, which gives the skin much of its elasticity and strength.

- *Subcutaneous Layer* -- Beneath the dermis lays the final layer of skin, the subcutaneous layer. The most notable structures here are the large groupings of adipose tissue. The main function of the subcutaneous layer is therefore to provide a cushion for the delicate organs lying beneath the skin. It also functions to insulate the body to maintain body temperature.

Vascular System

Layers of the heart -- Three layers of tissue form the heart wall. The outer layer of the heart wall is the epicardium, the middle layer is the myocardium, and the inner layer is the endocardium.

- Epicardium- the membrane that covers the outside of the heart
- Myocardium-The muscular wall of the heart, the thickest of the three layers of the heart wall, it lies between the inner layer (endocardium) and the outer layer (epicardium).
- Endocardium- membrane lining the inside surface of heart

Cardiac cycle

- Ventricular Systole:
  - Ventricles contract
  - Ventricular contraction regulated by AV node
  - Semilunar valves (to aorta & pulmonary arteries) open
  - Atrioventricular valves close ("lub")
- Ventricular Diastole:
  - Ventricles relax, atria contract
  - Atrial contraction regulated by SA node (pacemaker)
  - Semilunar valves close ("dupp")
  - Atrioventricular valves open

Origin of heart sounds (the heart beat)

A heartbeat is a two-part pumping action that takes about a second. As blood collects in the upper chambers (the right and left atria), the heart's natural pacemaker (the SA node) sends out an electrical signal that causes the atria to contract. This contraction pushes blood through the tricuspid and mitral valves into the resting lower chambers (the right and left ventricles). This part of the two-part pumping phase (the longer of the two) is called the diastole. The second part of the pumping phase begins when the ventricles are full of blood. The electrical signals from the SA node travel along a pathway of cells to the ventricles, causing them to contract. This is called systole. As the tricuspid and mitral valves shut tight to prevent a back flow of blood; the pulmonary and aortic valves are pushed open. While blood is pushed from the right ventricle into the lungs to pick up oxygen, oxygen-rich blood flows from the left ventricle to the heart and other parts of the body. After blood moves into the pulmonary artery and the aorta, the ventricles relax, and the pulmonary and aortic valves close. The lower pressure in the ventricles causes the tricuspid and mitral valves to open, and the cycle begins again. This series of contractions is repeated over and over again, increasing during times of exertion and decreasing while at rest.

Heart rate, cardiac output, and stroke volume

- *Heart Rate* -- The number of contractions of the heart in one minute. It is measured in beats per minute (bpm). When resting, the adult human heart beats at about 70 bpm (males) and 75 bpm (females), but this rate varies between people.
- *Cardiac output* -- The volume of blood being pumped by the heart in a minute. It is equal to the heart rate multiplied by the stroke volume.
- *Stroke Volume* -- The amount of blood ejected by the ventricle of the heart with each beat, usually expressed in milliliters (ml).

Electrical Conduction System

Electrical impulses from your heart muscle (the myocardium) cause your heart to beat (contract). This electrical signal begins in the sinoatrial (SA) node, located at the top of the right atrium. The SA node is sometimes called the heart's "natural pacemaker." When an electrical impulse is released from this natural pacemaker, it causes the atria to contract. The signal then passes through the atrioventricular (AV) node. The AV node checks the signal and sends it through the muscle fibers of the ventricles, causing them to contract. The SA node sends electrical impulses at a certain rate, but your heart rate may still change depending on physical demands, stress or hormonal factors.

The main functions of the vascular system include:

- Transport of materials
  - Gases transported -- Oxygen is transported from the lungs to the cells. CO_2 (a waste) is transported from the cells to the lungs.
  - Transport other nutrients to cells -- For example, glucose, a simple sugar used to produce ATP is transported throughout the body by the circulatory system. Immediately after digestion, glucose is transported to the liver. The liver maintains a constant level of glucose in the blood.

- Transport other wastes from cells -- For example, ammonia is produced as a result of protein digestion. It is transported to the liver where it is converted to less toxic urea. Urea is then transported to the kidneys for excretion in the urine.
- Transport hormones -- Numerous hormones that help maintain constant internal conditions are transported by the vascular system.
- Contains cells that fight infection
- Helps stabilize the pH and ionic concentration of the body fluids.
- It helps maintain body temperature by transporting heat.

Pulse and blood pressure
- *Pulse* -- The expansion and contraction of a blood vessel due to the blood pumped through it; determined as the number of expansions per minute
- *Blood Pressure* -- The force exerted in the arteries by blood as it circulates. It is divided into systolic (when the heart contracts) and diastolic (when the heart is filling) pressures

Blood vessels
- *Arteries* -- Blood vessels that carry blood away from the heart to the body, does not have valves
- *Veins* -- Blood vessels that carry the blood from the body back to the heart, has valves
- *Capillaries* – One cell thick blood vessels between arteries and veins that distribute oxygen-rich blood to the body
- *Venules* -- The smallest veins
- *Arterioles* -- The smallest arteries.

Wall of an artery consists of three (3) distinct layers of tunics
- Tunica intima -- Composed of simple, squamous epithelium called endothelium. Rests on a connective tissue membrane that is rich in elastic and collagenous fibers.
- Tunica media -- Makes up the bulk of the arterial wall. Includes smooth muscle fibers, which encircle the tube, and a thick layer of elastic connective tissue.

- Tunica adventitia -- Consists chiefly of connective tissue with irregularly arranged elastic and collagenous fibers. This layer attaches the artery to the surrounding tissues. Also contains minute vessels (vasa vasorum--vessels of vessels) that give rise to capillaries and provide blood to the more external cells of the artery wall.

Smooth muscles in the walls of arteries and arterioles are innervated by the sympathetic branches of the autonomic nervous system. The Tunica media and the Tunica adventitia are much thicker in arteries.

Chosing the best vein for venipuncture between the cubital, the basilica, and cephalic veins

First choice would be the median cubital due to its large size, and it usually doesn't bruise severely. Next choice would be the cephalic vein since it does not roll as easily as other veins. A last resort vein would be the basilica vein because it rolls easily and is positioned so that the brachial artery and a major nerve are at risk for puncture if used. Ankle and foot veins should only be punctured at the discretion of a physician and should only be used when no other veins are appropriate. Poor circulation and clotting factors may affect results of tests and cause puncture wounds that may not readily heal.

Lumen and valve

- *Lumen* -- The hollow area within a blood vessel
- *Valves* -- Tissue flaps inside a vein or the heart that prevent backward flow of blood. Valves open as blood moves through them and close under the weight of blood collecting in the vein due to decreased pressure and gravity.

Functions of the blood and blood components

Blood has numerous functions – gas transport, haemostasis, defence against disease – all of which are brought about by its various components:

- *Red blood cells* -- Oxygen transport and gas exchange
- Blood platelets and coagulation factors – coagulation and haemostasis
- *Vitamin K* -- Essential cofactor in normal hepatic synthesis of some clotting factors
- *Plasmin* -- Lyses fibrin and fibrinogen
- *Antithrombin III* -- Inhibits IXa, Xa, XIa, XIIa,
- *Complement* -- Defence against pyogenic bacteria, activation of phagocytes, clearing of immune complexes, lytic attack on cell membranes

- *Lymphocytes* -- Adaptive immune response – killing of specific microbes
- *Monocytes* -- Respond to necrotic cell material by migrating to tissues and differentiating into macrophages
- *Neutrophils* -- Phagocytosis of microbes
- *Eosinophils* -- Phagocytosis, defence against helminthic parasites, allergic reactions
- *Basophils* -- Allergic reactions

<u>Location of the Great saphenous, popliteal, femoral, lesser saphenous veins</u>:
- *Great saphenous* -- Runs the entire length of the lower extremity and is the longest vein in the body
- *Popliteal* -- Runs deep behind the knee
- *Femoral* -- Runs deep in the upper part of the leg
- *Lesser saphenous* -- Runs lateral to the ankle, up the leg and deep behind the knee

<u>Forces that move blood in the circulatory system through arteries vs. veins</u>
The blood flowing through the arterial system is pushed by the pressure built up by the contractions of the heart. The blood flowing through the veins relies on skeletal muscle movement to keep the valves located in the veins opening and closing to keep blood moving towards the heart and not backwards through the system.

<u>Irregularities</u>
- *Extrasystole* -- A premature systole resulting in a momentary cardiac arrhythmia referred to as an extra heart beat
- *Fibrillation* -- Rapid, inefficient contraction of muscle fibers of the heart caused by disruption of nerve impulses
- *Arrhythmia* -- An abnormal rate of muscle contractions in the heart which can present as bradycardia(too slow), tachycardia (too fast) or irregular
- *Murmur* -- The noise between normal heart sounds caused by blood flow through a heart valve

<u>Anemia</u>
Anaemia refers to any condition where there is reduced oxygen carrying capacity due to a fall in haemoglobin concentration with resultant tissue hypoxia. It is defined as Hb less than 13.5g/dl in males, <11/5g/dl in females, <15g/dl in newborns to three month olds, and less than 11g/dl from three months to puberty.

Anaemia results when compensatory mechanisms fail to restore oxygen levels to meet tissue demands. The following compensatory mechanisms are seen – arteriolar dilatation, increased cardiac output, increased anaerobic metabolism, increased Hb dissociation, increased erythropoietin output, and internal redistribution of blood flow. If these compensatory mechanisms are adequate, oxygen levels are restored. If not, anaemia ensues, with cardiac effects, poor exercise tolerance, lethargy, pallor, headaches, angina on effort and claudication.

Skeletal cells

Functional characteristics of a skeletal muscle cell
The cell membrane is called the sarcolemma. This membrane is structured to receive and conduct stimuli. The sarcoplasm of the cell is filled with contractile myofibrils and this results in the nuclei and other organelles being relegated to the edge of the cell.

Myofibrils are contractile units within the cell which consist of a regular array of protein myofilaments. Each myofilament runs longitudinally with respect to the muscle fiber. There are two types: the thick bands and the thin bands. Thick bands are made of multiple molecules of a protein called myosin.

The thin bands are made of multiple molecules of a protein called actin. The thin actin bands are attached to a Z-line or Z-disk of an elastic protein called titin. The titin protein also extends into the myofibril anchoring the other bands in position. From each Z-line to the next is a unit called the sarcomere.

Bone Cells
The cells of bone are osteocytes, osteoblasts, and osteoclasts.
- *Osteocytes* are found singly in lacunae (spaces) within the calcified matrix and communicate with each other via small canals in the bone known as canaliculi. The latter contain osteocyte cell processes. The osteocytes in compact and spongy bone are similar in structure and function.
- *Osteoblasts* are cells which form bone matrix, surrounding themselves with it, and thus are transformed into osteocytes. They arise from undifferentiated cells, such as mesenchymal cells. They are cuboidal cells which line the trabeculae of immature or developing spongy bone.

- *Osteoclasts* are cells found during bone development and remodeling. Osteoclasts remove the existing calcified matrix releasing the inorganic or organic components.

Arteries of the upper limb
- *Internal thoracic* -- Descends posterior to sternal end of clavicle and enters thorax
- *Thyrocervical trunk* -- Ascends as short trunk, gives off four branches; transverse and ascending cervical, suprascapular
- *Suprascapular* -- Passes inferolaterally, runs parallel to clavicle, then passes posteriorly to scapula
- *Subscapular* -- Descends along lateral border of subscapularis to inferior angle of scapula
- *Thoracodorsal* -- Accompanies thoracodorsal nerve to latissimus dorsi
- *Deep Brachial* -- Accompanies radial nerve through radial groove in humerus, anastamoses around elbow joint
- *Ulnar Collateral* -- Both anastamose around elbow joint

Key nerves of the arm
- *Musculocutaneous Nerve* -- Supplies all the muscles in the anterior (flexor) compartment of the arm, In the interval between the biceps and brachialis it becomes the lateral cutaneous nerve of forearm which supplies a large area of forearm skin.
- *Radial Nerve* -- Supplies all the muscles in the posterior compartment of the arm, Descends inferolaterally with deep brachial artery around humerus in radial groove, Divides into deep and superficial branches:
  o Deep Branch (entirely muscular in distribution)
  o Superficial Branch (entirely cutaneous, supply dorsum of hand and digits)
- *Median Nerve* -- No branches in arm, Runs initially on lateral side of brachial artery, crosses it at middle of arm Descends to cubital fossa deep to bicipital aponeurosis.
- Ulnar Nerve -- No branches in arm, Passes anterior to triceps on medial side of brachial artery, Passes posterior to medial epicondyle and medial to olecranon to enter forearm.

Meaning of an ECG tracing of a cardiac cycle

- P wave represent the atrial depolarization
- QRS complex represents the Ventricular depolarization
- T wave represents the ventricular repolarization

Relationship between plasma K+ and arterial pH

Cells exchange K+ and H+ with plasma. In metabolic acidosis, plasma K+ concentration increases, even though body potassium may become depleted. In metabolic alkalosis, plasma K+ concentration may decrease. But although cells gain K+ initially, chronic alkalosis may result in loss of body potassium because of increased K+ excretion by renal principal cells due to increased Na+ delivery to this segment encouraging exchange of Na+ for cell K+ with K+ staying in the lumen to maintain electroneutrality. Chronic K+ depletion can result in alkalosis where decreased K+ secretion by depleted principal cells results in a greater portion of the Na+ delivered to the distal tubule being reabsorbed in exchange for secreted H+ ions. The corresponding transfer of cell HCO_3- to the plasma may explain the paradoxical association of an acid urine with an alkaline plasma.

Terms oxygenation and oxidation as applied to haemoglobin

Oxygenation is the loose, reversible binding of Hb with O2 molecules forming oxyHb. Hb oxygenation is the principle method of O2 uptake from the lungs into the RBCs for transport to the tissues.

Each Hb molecule has the capacity to bind four O2 molecules since there are four haem molecules in each Hb. O2 binds loosely with the co-ordination bonds of the iron atom in the haem and not the two positive bonds of the iron. Iron is not oxidized and oxygen can be carried to the tissues in the molecular form rather than the ionic form.

Oxidation of Hb involves the conversion of the functional ferrous ($Fe2+$) haem iron to the non-functional ferric ($Fe3+$) form. This is called methaemoglobin. This oxidized form of Hb can't bind or transport oxygen. Oxidation of Hb may occur due to exposure to toxic chemicals such as nitrites, aniline dyes and oxidative drugs.

Immunoglobulin

Types of immunoglobulin and their functions:
- IgA– can be located in secretions and prevents viral and bacterial attachment to membranes.
- IgD- can be located on B cells
- IgE-main mediator of mast cells with allergen exposure.
- IgG- primarily found in secondary responses. Does cross placenta and destroys viruses/bacteria.
- IgM- primarily found in first response. Located on B cells

Testing aldosterone levels

Aldosterone is an adrenal hormone. It has a role in the regulation of water and sodium in the kidneys. A patient must be in the upright position for at least 30 minutes prior to the collection of the specimen. Also, the test is usually preformed in the chemistry department.

Cytomegalovirus

Abbreviated as CMV, Cytomegalovirus is a herpes virus which can result in a life threatening situation if an infant contracts it before it is born. It can cause pneumonia or in some children result in developmental delays. CMV is tested for by an immunology test performed on serum.

Lactic acid

Lactic acid is produced by glucose-burning cells when these cells have an inadequate supply of oxygen. Lactic acid is produced in excess as a result of an oxygen deficient state called hypoxia. Examples of hypoxia are shock, hypovolemia and left ventricle failure. Excess amounts can also be caused by diabetes mellitus and toxicity. Lactic acidosis is the state where there is too much lactic acid in the blood.

Important terms

Frontal (Coronal) Plane -- A plane parallel to the long axis of the body and perpendicular to the sagittal plane that separates the body into front and back portions.

Sagittal Plane -- A plane that divides the body into right and left halves

Transverse (Horizontal) Plane -- A plane that divides the body into upper and lower sections

Medical Terminology

Prefixes

A -- without
An -- without
Ante -- before
Bi -- two
Bin -- two
Brady -- slow
Dia -- through
Dys -- difficult
Endo -- within
Epi -- over
Eu -- normal
Ex -- outward
Exo -- outward
Hemi -- half
Hyper -- excessive
Hypo -- deficient
Inter -- between
Intra -- within
Meta -- change
Micro -- minute, tiny
Multi -- numerous
Neo -- new
Nulli -- none
Pan -- total
Para -- beyond
Per -- through
Peri -- surrounding
Poly -- many
Post -- after
Pre -- before
Pro -- before
Sub -- below

Supra -- superior
Sym -- join
Syn -- join
Tachy -- rapid
Tetra -- four
Trans -- through
Uni -- one

Suffixes

-ac -- pertaining to
-ad -- toward
-al -- pertaining to
-algia -- pain
-apheresis -- removal
-ar -- pertaining to
-ary -- pertaining to
-asthenia -- weakness
-atresia -- occlusion, closure
-capnia -- carbon dioxide
-cele -- hernia
-centesis -- aspirate fluid off lung
-clasia -- break
-clasis -- break
-coccus -- berry-like bacteria
-crit -- separate
-cyte -- cell
-desis -- fusion
-drome -- run
-eal -- pertaining to
-ectasis -- expansion
-ectomy -- removal
-emia -- blood dysfunction
-esis -- condition
-gen -- agent that causes
-genesis -- cause
-genic -- pertaining to
-gram -- record

-graph -- recording device

-graphy -- process of recording

-ia -- disease condition

-ial -- pertaining to

-iasis -- condition

-iatrist -- physician

-iatry -- specialty

-ic -- pertaining to

-ician -- one that

-ictal -- attack

-ior -- pertaining to

-ism -- condition of

-it is -- inflammation

-lysis -- separating

-malacia -- softening

-megaly -- increasing in size

-meter -- measure

-odynia -- pain

-oid -- resembling

-ologist -- person that practices

-ology -- study

-oma -- tumor

-opia -- vision

-opsy -- view of

-orrhagia -- blood flowing profusely

-orrhaphy -- repairing

-orrhea -- flow

-orrhexis -- break

-osis -- condition

-ostomy -- to make an opening

-otomy -- cut into

-ous -- pertaining to

-oxia -- oxygen

-paresis -- partial paralysis

-pathy -- disease

-penia -- decrease in number

-pepsia -- digestion

-pexy -- suspension

-phagia -- swallowing, eating

-phobia -- excessive fear of

-phonia -- sound, voice

-physis -- growth

-plasia -- development

-plasm -- a growth

-plasty -- repair by surgery

-plegia -- paralysis

-pnea -- breathing

-poiesis -- formation

-ptosis -- sagging

-salpinx -- fallopian tube

-sarcoma -- malignant tumor

-schisis -- crack

-sclerosis -- hardening

-scope -- visual device used for inspection

-scopic -- visual inspection

-sis -- condition of

-spasm -- abnormal muscle firing

-stasis -- standing

-stenosis -- narrowing

-thorax -- chest

-tocia -- labor, birth

-tome -- cutting device

-tripsy -- surgical crushing

-trophy -- develop

-uria -- urine

Word roots

abdomin/o -- abdomen

acou/o -- hearing

acr/o -- height/extremities

aden/o -- gland

adenoid/o -- adenoids

adren/o -- adrenal gland

alveol/o -- alveolus

amni/o -- amnion

andro/o -- male

angi/o -- vessel

ankly/o -- stiff

anter/o -- frontal

an/o -- anus

aponeur/o -- aponeurosis

appendic/o -- appendix

arche/o -- beginning

arteri/o -- artery

athero/o -- fatty plaque

atri/o -- atrium

aur/I -- ear

aur/o -- ear

aut/o -- self

azot/o -- nitrogen

bacteri/o -- bacteria

balan/o   glans penis

bi/o -- life

blast/o -- developing cell

blephar/o -- eyelid

bronch/I -- bronchus

bronch/o -- bronchus

burs/o -- bursa

calc/I -- calcium

cancer/o -- cancer

carcin/o -- cancer

cardi/o -- heart

carp/o -- carpals

caud/o -- tail

cec/o -- cecum

celi/o -- abdomen

cephal/o -- head

cerebell/o -- cerebellum

cerebr/o -- cerebrum

cervic/o -- cervix

cheil/o   -- lip

cholangi/o -- bile duct

chol/e -- gall

- 23 -

chondro/o -- cartilage

chori/o -- chorion

chrom/o -- color

clavic/o -- clavicle

clavicul/o -- clavicle

col/o -- colon

colp/o -- vagina

core/o -- pupil

corne/o -- cornea

coron/o -- heart

cortic/o -- cortex

cor/o -- pupil

cost/o -- rib

crani/o -- cranium

cry/o -- cold

cutane/o -- skin

cyan/o   -- blue

cyes/i -- pregnancy

cyst/o -- bladder

cyt/o -- cell

dacry/o -- tear

dermat/o -- skin

derm/o -- skin

diaphragmat/o -- diaphragm

dipl/o -- double

dips/o -- thirst

disk/o -- disk

dist/o -- distal

diverticul/o -- diverticulum

dors/o -- back

duoden/o -- duodenum

dur/o -- dura

ech/o -- sound

electr/o -- electricity

embry/o -- embryo

encephal/o -- brain

endocrin/o -- endocrine

enter/o -- intestine

epididym/o -- epididymis
epiglott/o -- epiglottis
episi/o -- vulva
epitheli/o -- epithelium
erythr/o -- red
esophag/o -- esophagus
esthesi/o -- sensation
eti/o -- cause of disease
femor/o -- femur
fet/I - fetus
fet/o -- fetus
fibr/o -- fibrous tissue
fibul/o -- fibula
gangli/o -- ganglion
ganglion/o -- ganglion
gastr/o -- stomach
gingiv/o -- gum
glomerul/o -- glomerulus
gloss/o -- tongue
glyc/o -- sugar
gnos/o -- knowledge
gravid/o -- pregnancy
gynec/o -- woman
gyn/o -- woman
hem/o -- blood
hemat/o -- blood
hepat/o -- liver
herni/o -- hernia
heter/o   other
hidr/o -- sweat
hist/o -- tissue
humer/o -- humerus
hydr/o -- water
hymen/o -- hymen
hyster/o -- uterus
ile/o -- ileum
ili/o -- ilium
infer/o -- inferior

irid/o -- iris
iri/o -- iris
ischi/o -- ischium
ischo/o -- blockage
jejun/o -- jejunum
kal/I -- potassium
kary/o-- nucleus
kerat/o -- hard
kinesi/o -- motion
kyph/o -- hump
lacrim/o -- tear duct
lact/o -- milk
lamin/o -- lamina
lapar/o -- abdomen
laryng/o -- larynx
later/o -- lateral
lei/o -- smooth
leuk/o -- white
lingu/o -- tongue
lip/o -- fat
lith/o -- stone
lord/o -- flexed forward
lumb/o -- lumbar
lymph/o -- lymph
mamm/o -- breast
mandibul/o -- mandible
mast/o -- breast
mastoid/o -- mastoid
maxill/o -- maxilla
meat/o -- opening
melan/o -- black
mening/o -- meninges
menisc/o -- meniscus
men/o -- menstruation
ment/o -- mind
metr/I -- uterus
metr/o-- uterus
mon/o-- one

muc/o -- mucus

myc/o -- fungus

myel/o -- spinal cord

myelon/o -- bone marrow

myos/o -- muscle

my/o -- muscle

nas/o -- nose

nat/o -- birth

necr/o -- death

nephr/o -- kidney

neur/o -- nerve

noct/I -- night

ocul/o -- eye

olig/o -- few

omphal/o -- navel

onc/o -- tumor

onych/o -- nail

oophor/o -- ovary

ophthalm/o -- eye

opt/o -- vision

orchid/o -- testicle

orch/o -- testicle

organ/o -- organ

or/o -- mouth

orth/o -- straight

oste/o -- bone

ot/o -- ear

ox/I -- oxygen

pachy/o -- thick

palat/o -- palate

pancreat/o -- pancreas

parathyroid/o-- parathyroid gland

par/o -- labor

patell/o -- patella

path/o-- disease

pelv/I -- pelvis

perine/o -- peritoneum

petr/o -- stone

phalang/o -- pharynx

phas/o -- speech

phleb/o -- vein

phot/o -- light

phren/o -- mind

plasm/o -- plasma

pleur/o -- pleura

pneumat/o -- lung

pneum/o -- lung

pneumon/o -- lung

poli/o -- gray matter

polyp/o -- small growth

poster/o -- posterior

prim/I -- first

proct/o -- rectum

prostat/o -- prostate gland

proxim/o -- proximal

pseud/o -- fake

psych/o -- mind

pub/o -- pubis

puerper/o -- childbirth

pulmon/o -- lung

pupill/o -- pupil

pyel/o -- renal pelvis

pylor/o -- pylorus

py/o -- pus

quadr/I -- four

rachi/o -- spinal

radic/o -- nerve

radicul/o -- nerve

radi/o -- radius

rect/o -- rectum

ren/o -- kidney

retin/o -- retina

rhabd/o -- striated

rhin/o -- nose

rhytid/o -- wrinkles

rhiz/o -- nerve

salping/o -- fallopian tube

sacr/o -- sacrum

scapul/o -- scapula

scler/o -- sclera

scoli/o -- curved

seb/o -- sebum

sept/o -- septum

sial/o -- saliva

sinus/o -- sinus

somat/o -- body

son/o -- sound

spermat/o -- sperm

sphygm/o -- pulse

spir/o -- breathe

splen/o -- spleen

spondyl/o -- vertebra

staped/o -- stapes

staphyl/o -- clusters

stern/o -- sternum

steth/o -- chest

stomat/o -- mouth

strept/o -- chain-like

super/o -- superior

synovi/o -- synovia

system/o -- system

tars/o -- tarsal

tendin/o -- tendon

ten/o -- tendon

test/o -- testicle

therm/o -- heat

thorac/o -- thorax

thromb/o -- clot

thym/o -- thymus

thyroid/o -- thyroid gland

thyr/o -- thyroid gland

tibi/o -- tibia

tom/o -- pressure

tonsill/o -- tonsils

toxic/o -- poison

trachel/o -- trachea

trich/o -- hair

tympan/o -- eardrum

uln/o -- ulna

ungu/o -- nail

ureter/o -- ureter

urethr/o -- urethra

urin/o -- urine

ur/o -- urine

uter/o -- uterus

uvul/o -- uvula

vagin/o -- vagina

valv/o -- valve

valvul/o -- valve

vas/o -- vessel

ven/o -- vein

ventricul/o -- ventricle

ventro/o -- frontal

vertebr/o -- vertebra

vesic/o -- bladder

vesicul/o -- seminal vesicles

viscer/o -- internal organs

vulv/o -- vulva

xanth/o -- yellow

xer/o -- dry

Abbreviations

Autonomic nervous system -- ANS

Anterior -- ant

As soon as possible -- ASAP

Arteriovenous -- AV

Twice a day -- bid

Blood pressure -- BP

Beats per minute -- bpm

Blood urea nitrogen -- BUN

Biopsy -- Bx

Culture and sensitivity -- C&S

Calcium -- Ca

Completer blood count -- CBC

Colony count -- CC

Carcinoma embryonic antigen -- CEA

Chloride -- Cl

Central nervous system -- CNS

Creatine phosphokinase -- CPK

Cardiopulmonary resuscitation -- CPR

Cerebrospinal fluid -- CSF

Cardiovascular -- CV

Central venous pressure -- CVP

Discharge -- D/C

Distilled water -- DW

Diagnosis -- Dx

Estimated blood loss -- EBL

In the manner prescribed -- e.m.p.

Estrogen replacement therapy - ERT

Erythrocyte sedimentation rate - ESR

Etiology -- etiol

Fasting blood sugar -- FBS

Iron -- Fe

Follicle-stimulating hormone -- FSH

Gram -- g

Gastroesophageal reflux disease -- GERD

Gradually -- Grad.

Glucose tolerance test -- GTT

Hour -- h

Hypodermic -- H or hypo.

Hemodialysis- HD

Hemoglobin and hematocrit -- H&H

Hematocrit -- Hct

Mercury -- Hg

Hemoglobin- Hgb

Human immunodeficiency virus -- HIV

History and physical -- H&P

Intramuscular -- IM

Intravenous -- IV

Potassium -- K

Potassium Chloride -- KCL

Keep Vein Open -- KVO

Laboratory --lab

Medications -- meds

Multiple Sclerosis -- MS

Sodium -- Na

Newborn -- NB

Negative -- neg

NPO -- nothing by mouth

Oxygen -- O_2

Overdose -- OD

After meals - pc

Packed Cell Volume -- PCV

Between noon and midnight --PM

Positive -- pos.

Postoperatively --post-op

Packed Red Blood Cells -- PRBC

Prostatic specific antigen -- PSA

Prothrombin time -- PT

Physical Therapy -- PT

Every day -- qd

Every other day -- qod

Immediately -- stat

Three times a day – tid

RAST

RAST is an abbreviation for the radioallergosorbent test. This test is used in the detection of allergies for example a peanut allergy.

@@@
Tumor markers

A tumor marker is a substance sometimes found in the blood, other body fluids, or tissues. A high level of tumor marker may indicate that a certain type of cancer is in the body. Examples of tumor markers include CA 125 (ovarian cancer), CA 15-3 (breast cancer), CEA (ovarian, lung, breast, pancreas, and gastrointestinal tract

- 32 -

cancers), and PSA (prostate cancer). Tumor makers are sometimes called biomarker.

Fahrenheit and Celcius

Fahrenheit into Celcius
C = (F - 32) x 5/9
Celsius into Fahrenheit
F = (C x 9/5) + 32

Roman numerals

The following Roman numerals equal the Arabic numbers.
- I = 1
- V = 5
- X = 10
- L = 50
- C = 100
- D = 500
- M = 1000

Blood culture dilution

The dilution of 1:100 means that there is 1mL of blood and 99mL of media for every 100 mL of blood culture specimen.

Fahrenheit and Celsius degrees

Normal body temperature 98.6°F 37°C
Room temperature 68-77°F 20-25°C
Boiling point of water 212°F   100°C
Freezing point of water 32°F   0°C

Approximating liters of blood

Liters of blood in adults
The average adult has 70 mL of blood per kilogram of weight. In the United States, a person weigh is usually recorded in pounds. You will need to convert the pounds

into kilograms by using the conversion factor of 0.454. The person's weight in kilograms is multiplied by 70 which is the average mL of blood per kilogram. Then divide that number by 1000 to convert the mL into Liters.

<u>Liters of blood in infants</u>

The average infant has 100 mL of blood per kilogram of weight. If an infant's weight is given in pounds it must be converted to kilograms using the conversion factor of 0.454. That number is then multiplied by 100 which is the average mL of blood per kilogram in an infant. Then divide that number by 1000 to convert the mL into liters.

Important terms

Gram -- basic metric unit of weight
Meter -- basic metric unit of distance
Liter -- basic metric unit of volume

Important Formulas

(amount ÷ total) × 100 = percentage
Kilograms = (Pounds x 0.4536)

	Metric	English
Distance	meter	3.3 feet
Weight	gram	.0022 pounds
Volume	liter	1.06 quarts

Military to civilian time

Military = Civilian	Military = Civilian
0001 = 12:01 AM	1200 = 12 Noon
0100 = 1:00 AM	1300 = 1:00 PM
0200 = 2:00 AM	1400 = 2:00 PM
0300 = 3:00 AM	1500 = 3:00 PM
0400 = 4:00 AM	1600 = 4:00 PM
0500 = 5:00 AM	1700 = 5:00 PM
0600 = 6:00 AM	1800 = 6:00 PM
0700 = 7:00 AM	1900 = 7:00 PM
0800 = 8:00 AM	2000 = 8:00 PM
0900 = 9:00 AM	2100 = 9:00 PM
1000 = 10:00 AM	2200 = 10:00 PM
1100 = 11:00 AM	2300 = 11:00 PM
1200 = 12 Noon	0000 = 12 Midnight

Professional Behavior, Ethics, and Legal Issues

Patient consent -- The types of patient consents needed to do a proceedure:

- *Informed Consent* -- A competent person gives voluntary permission for a medical procedure after receiving adequate information about the risk of, methods used and consequences of the procedure
- *Expressed Consent* -- Permission given by patient verbally or in writing for a procedure
- *Implied Consent* -- The patient's actions gives permission for the procedure without verbal or written consent for example going to the emergency room or holding out arm when told need to draw blood.
- *HIV Consent* -- Special permission given to administer a test for detecting the human immunodeficiency virus.
- *Parental Consent for Minors* -- A parent or a legal guardian must give permission for procedures administered to underage patients depending on the state law may range from 18 to 21 years old.

Dr. W. Edwards Deming

Deming is the Father of Quality Evolution. The following are the points that he believed would improve quality assurance:

- Create and communicate to all employees a statement of the aims and purposes of the company.
- Adapt to the new philosophy of the day; industries and economics are always changing.
- Build quality into a product throughout production.
- End the practice of awarding business on the basis of price tag alone; instead, try a long-term relationship based on established loyalty and trust.
- Work to constantly improve quality and productivity.
- Institute on-the-job training.
- Teach and institute leadership to improve all job functions.
- Drive out fear; create trust.
- Strive to reduce intradepartmental conflicts.
- Eliminate exhortations for the work force; instead, focus on the system and morale.

- Eliminate work standard quotas for production. Substitute leadership methods for improvement.
- Eliminate MBO.
- Avoid numerical goals. Alternatively, learn the capabilities of processes, and how to improve them.
- Remove barriers that rob people of pride of workmanship.
- Educate with self-improvement programs.
- Include everyone in the company to accomplish the transformation.

Agencies

The following agencies' responsibilities are:
- <u>National Accrediting Agency for Clinical Laboratory Sciences</u> -- Agency for accreditation and approval of education programs in the clinical laboratory sciences and related health care professions
- <u>National Committee for Clinical Laboratory Standards</u> -- Standards-developing organization that promotes the development and use of voluntary consensus standards and guidelines within the healthcare community
- <u>College of American Pathologist</u> -- The principal organization of board-certified pathologists that serves and represents the interests of patients, pathologists, and the public by fostering excellence in the practice of pathology and laboratory medicine.
- <u>Joint Commission on Accreditation of Healthcare Organizations</u> -- organization that strives to continuously improve the safety and quality of care provided to the public through the provision of health care accreditation and related services that support performance improvement in health care organizations

Patient rights

The following situations violate patient's rights:
- *A patient is told that he will be restrained if he doesn't stop moving so that a specimen can be collected.* The patient has been threatened with the fear of restraint. This falls into the category of assault.
- *A co-worker tells you that your patient, Mr. Louis, has HIV in the hospital cafeteria.* This is a breach of confidentiality. The information has been given to you in an inappropriate location. Someone who knows Mr. Louis may have

overheard the information exchange. All information about a patient should be considered confidential.

- *An unsupervised 10-year old refuses to have his blood drawn; a co-worker helps hold him down while you draw the blood.* If the parents are not there to consent to a blood draw, this may be considered assault and battery.
- *You forget to put a needle in the sharp's container and a 2 year old gets stuck.* This is a case of negligence. You were responsible for putting the needle into the sharp's container and harm was done to the child as a result of your action.

Important terms

Tort -- An injury or wrong committed, either with or without force, to the person or property of another, for which civil liability may be imposed.

Assault -- The touching of another person with intent to harm, without that person's consent, A willful attempt to illegally inflict injury on or threaten a person

Malpractice -- A lawsuit brought against a professional person for injury or loss caused by the defendant's negligence in providing professional services

Negligence -- Failure to act with the prudence that a reasonable person would exercise under the same circumstances

Vicarious liability -- When a person is held responsible for the tort of another even though the person being held responsible may not have done anything wrong. This is often the case with employers who are held vicariously liable for the damages caused by their employees.

Breach of Confidentiality -- Occurs when information that should be kept secret, with access limited to appropriate persons, is given to an inappropriate person

Fraud -- An intentional perversion of truth; deceitful practice or device resorted to with intent to deprive another of property or other right.

Risk Management -- System that involves identifying and reducing situations that pose unnecessary risk to employees or patients by following specific procedures and by adequately educating employees on policies and procedures adopted by the facility.

Quality Control -- A series of checks and control measures that ensure that a uniform excellence of service is provided

Quality Assurance -- Activities involving a review of quality of services and the taking of any corrective actions to remove or improve any deficiencies

Infection Control and Safety

Hazards route into body

The following are ways biological hazards enter the human body:
- Airborne (through the nasal passage into the lungs)
- Ingestion (by eating)
- Broken Skin
- Percutaneous (through intact skin)
- Mucosal (through the lining of the mouth and nose)

Infection Control Methods

The first line of defense in infection control is hand washing. Protective Clothing is an important aspect of infection control. This includes Masks, Goggles, Face Shields, Respirators, Gowns, Lab Coats, and Gloves. The precautions that are used depend on the infection. Isolation procedures are also used this includes protective isolation or reverse isolation. In protective isolation, the patients are isolated to prevent them from getting an infection i.e. patients receiving chemotherapy. In reverse isolation, the patients are isolated to prevent others from getting their infection or disease i.e. patients with tuberculosis. Universal Precautions are used with all patients. This means do not touch or use anything that has the patient's body fluid on it without a barrier and assume that all body fluid of a patient is infectious.

Hepatitis D Virus

Hepatitis D Virus is usually acquired with HBV as a co-infection or super infection:
- *Signs and Symptoms* -- jaundice, fatigue, abdominal pain, loss of appetite, nausea, vomiting, joint pain, dark (tea colored) urine
- *Transmission* -- Occurs when blood from an infected person enters the body of a person who is not immune; sharing drugs, needles, or "works" when "shooting" drugs; through needle sticks or sharps exposures on the job; or from an infected mother to her baby during birth.

- *Treatment*
  - Acute HDV infection -- Supportive care
  - Chronic HDV infection -- Interferon-alfa, liver transplant
- *Prevention*:
  - Hepatitis B vaccination
  - HBV-HDV co-infection
  - Pre- or post-exposure prophylaxis (hepatitis B immune globulin or vaccine) to prevent HBV infection
  - HBV-HDV superinfection
  - Education to reduce risk behaviors among persons with chronic HBV infection

Hepatitis B Virus

Sexually transmitted disease, also transmitted with body fluids and some individual may be symptom free but still be carriers. Condoms are not proved to prevent the spread of this disease. HBV is the most common laboratory-associated infection.

- *Symptoms* -- Jaundice, Dark Urine, Malaise, Joint pain, Fever, Fatigue
- *Tests* -- Decreased albumin levels, + antibodies and antigen; increased levels of transaminase
- *Treatment* -- Monitor for changes in the liver; recombinant alpha interferon in some cases; transplant necessary if liver failure occurs.
- *Prevention* -- Series of 3 Hepatitis B Vaccinations: an initial dose, a dose 1 month later and a final dose 6 months after the initial dose.

Communicable versus nosocomial Infections

Communicable Infection -- An illness due to a specific infectious agent or its toxic products that arises through transmission of that agent or its products from an infected person, animal or inanimate reservoir to a susceptible host; either directly or indirectly through an intermediate plant or animal host, vector or the inanimate environment (synonym: infectious disease)
Nosocomial Infection -- Illnesses acquired in the hospital inpatient environment not resulting from the reasons the patient was admitted

HIV transmission

Ways that HIV can be transmitted from an infected person to an uninfected one:

- *Unprotected sexual contact* -- Direct blood contact, including injection drug needles, blood transfusions, accidents in health care settings or certain blood products. Mother to baby (before or during birth, or through breast milk)
- *Sexual intercourse (vaginal and anal)* -- In the genitals and the rectum, HIV may infect the mucous membranes directly or enter through cuts and sores caused during intercourse (many of which would be unnoticed).
- *Oral sex (mouth-penis, mouth-vagina)* -- The mouth is an inhospitable environment for HIV (in semen, vaginal fluid or blood), meaning the risk of HIV transmission through the throat, gums, and oral membranes is lower than through vaginal or anal membranes. There are however, documented cases where HIV was transmitted orally.
- *Sharing injection needles* -- An injection needle can pass blood directly from one person's bloodstream to another. It is a very efficient way to transmit a blood-borne virus.
- *Mother to Child* -- It is possible for an HIV-infected mother to pass the virus directly before or during birth, or through breast milk. The following "bodily fluids" are NOT infectious: Saliva, Tears, Sweat, Feces, Urine

Cleaning blood spills

The best way to clean a small blood spill is to absorb the blood with a paper towel or gauze pad. Then disinfect area with a disinfectant. Soap and water is not a disinfectant nor is alcohol. Never scrape a dry spill; this may cause an aerosol of infectious organisms. If blood is dried, use the disinfectant to moisten the dried blood.

Fire safety

Fire requires three components to occur. They are called the fire triangle and include fuel, oxygen, and heat when a chemical source is included it forms the fire tetrahedron. In the event of a fire remember these two acronyms, RACE and PASS.

RACE describes the steps for dealing with a fire.

- "R" stands for Rescue (rescue patients and co-workers from danger.)
- "A" stands for alarm (sound the alarm and alert those around you.)
- "C" stands for confine (confine a fire by closing the doors and windows.)
- "E" stands for extinguish (use the nearest fire extinguisher to put out the fire.

PASS describes how to use a fire extinguisher to put out a fire.

- "P" stands for pull the pin.
- "A" stands for aim at the fire.
- "S" stands for squeeze the trigger.
- "S" stands for sweep the base of the fire. Fires are broken down into four classes.

Class A fires involve ordinary combustible materials. Class B fires involve flammable liquids, Class C involves electrical fires, and Class D involves combustible metals.

OSHA and SDS

OSHA stands for Occupational Safety and Health Administration. It is an organization designed to assure the safety and health of workers by setting and enforcing standards; providing training, outreach, and education; establishing partnerships; and encouraging continual improvement in workplace safety and health.

SDS, formerly MSDS, stands for Safety Data Sheets. These sheets are the result of the "Right to Know" Law also known as the OSHA's HazCom Standard. This law requires chemical manufacturers to supply SDSs on any products that have a hazardous warning label. These sheets contain information on precautionary as well as emergency information about the product.

Protective clothing

A healthcare worker puts on the protective gown first being sure not to touch the outside of the gown. The mask is put on next. Gloves are applied last and secured over the cuffs of the gown.

A healthcare worker removes the gloves first. They are removed by grasping one glove at the wrist and pulling it inside out off the hand and holding it in the gloved hand. The second glove is removed by placing your uncovered hands fingers under the edge of the glove being careful not to touch the outside of the glove and rolling it down inside out over the glove grasped in your hand. The first glove ends up inside of the second glove. Next, remove your mask by touching the strings only. Next slide your arms out of the gown and then fold the gown with the outside folded in away from your body so that the contaminated side is folded inwardly. Dispose of properly. Always wash hands after glove removal.

Equipment, Additives, and Order of Draw

Needle selection

The gauge of a needle is a number that is inversely correlates to the diameter of the internal space of the needle for example the larger the needle the smaller the internal space of the needle and the smaller the number the larger the internal space of the needle. Since color-coding varies between manufactures, be careful of using this method to determine the gauge of a needle. When selecting a needle for venipuncture, there are several factors to consider which include the type of procedure, the condition and size of the patient's vein, and the equipment being used. The length of the needle used is determined by the depth of the vein. Keep in mind that the smaller the gauge the larger the bore. The 21-gauge needle is the standard needle used for routine venipuncture.

Order of draw

Blood collection tubes must be drawn in a specific order to avoid cross-contamination of additives between tubes. The recommended order of draw is:
- *First* -- blood culture tube (yellow-black stopper)
- *Second* -- non-additive tube (red stopper or SST)
- *Third* -- coagulation tube (light blue stopper). If just a routine coagulation assay is the only test ordered, then a single light blue stopper tube may be drawn. If there is a concern regarding contamination by tissue fluids or thromboplastins, then one may draw a non-additive tube first, and then the light blue stopper.
- *Last draw* -- additive tubes in this order:
  - SST (red-gray, or gold, stopper). Contains a gel separator and clot activator.
  - Sodium heparin (dark green stopper)
  - PST (light green stopper). Contains lithium heparin anticoagulant and a gel separator.
  - EDTA (lavender stopper)
  - ACDA or ACDB (pale yellow stopper). Contains acid citrate dextrose.
  - Oxalate/fluoride (light gray stopper)

Disinfectants and antiseptics

Disinfectants are used to kill possible pathogens. They are bactericidal corrosive compounds composed of chemicals. Some disinfectants are capable of killing viruses such as HIV and HBV. These are not used on humans to disinfect skin. A common disinfectant is bleach in a 1:10 dilution. *Antiseptics* are chemical compounds that inhibit or prevent the growth of microorganism microbes usually applied externally. Antiseptics attempt to prevent sepsis but do not necessarily kill bacteria and viruses. Antiseptics are used on human skin. Common antiseptics include 70% isopropyl alcohol, betadine, and benzalkonium chloride with isopropyl alcohol being the most commonly used. Betadine is used when a sterile draw is needed.

Additives in colored stoppers

Yellow -- SPS and ACD
Red (glass tube) --no additive
Light blue -- sodium citrate
Lavender -- EDTA
Dark Green -- heparin
Gray -- potassium oxalate and sodium fluoride
Gold -- silica, thixotropic gel
Mottled red and gray -- silica, thixotropic gel

PPT, SST, and PST

All three tubes contain thixotropic gel which is a non-reactive synthetic substance that serves as an actual physical barrier between the serum and the cellular portion of a specimen after the specimen has been centrifuged. If thixotropic gel is used in tube with EDTA, it is referred to as a plasma preparation tube (PPT.) When thixotropic gel is used in serum collection tube, the gel is referred to as serum separator thus the tube and the gel are called the serum separator tube (SST.) When thixotropic gel is used in a tube with heparin, it is called plasma separator. Thus when thixotropic gel and heparin are in a tube; the tube is called the plasma separator tube (PST.)

Anticoagulants and antiglycolytic

Anticoagulant
EDTA
Citrates
Heparin
Oxalates

Antiglycolytic Agent
Sodium fluoride
Lithium iodoacetate

Tourniquets

A tourniquet is used to aid in the collection of a blood specimen. The tourniquet is tied in such a way that it is easily removed above the venipuncture site. The purpose of the tourniquet is to slow down venous flow away from the puncture site and to not inhibit arterial flow to the puncture site. By doing this, the vein enlarges to make it easier to locate and puncture. A tourniquet should not be left on longer than 1 minute because this may change the composition of the blood and make testing inaccurate.

Heparin

The anticoagulant heparin works by inhibiting thrombin which is required during the coagulation process. Thrombin is needed to form fibrin from fibrinogen. Thus when thrombin is inhibited a fibrin clot is less likely to develop.

Syringe system

Needle safety devices protect the needle user's hand by having it remain behind the needle during use and by providing a barrier between the user's hand and the needle after use. Also, the needle safety devices are operable with using a one-handed technique and provide a permanent barrier around the contaminated needle.

General comments

Concepts to remember:
- Adhesive bandages pose a choking hazard to children under the age of two.
- OSHA requires all sharps containers to be marked with a biohazard symbol.
- Household bleach this solution has been proven to kill HIV as well as HBV.
- Butterfly needles are used with infants and with difficult veins. 21-gauge needle is the standard needle used for routine venipuncture.

Important terms

Bevel – Slanted tip of a needle used to puncture the skin and vein without removing a piece of the vein.

Hub – End of a needle that attaches to the blood collection device i.e. syringe or tube holder.

Plunger – The part of the syringe that when pulled on creates a vacuum allowing the barrel of the syringe to be filled with fluid or air.

Shaft – The hollow round long cylinder-shaped part of a needle

Sharps container – An easily sealed, rigid, leak-proof, puncture-resistant, disposable box with a locking lid in which used needles and sharp materials are disposed.

Preparatory Steps, Site Selection, and Collection

Initiating patient contact

- Knock on door before entering patient's room, slowly open the door and ask if it is alright to enter.
- Look for signs on door indicating special precautions you need to take, i.e. protective clothing needed, your name and reason for entering room.
- In the event of a physician or member of the clergy being in the room, it is appropriate to explain who you are and proceed to do the draw if the draw is STAT.
- Ask the family to step out of the room.

Abbreviations

The following are important abbreviations and concepts for the phlebotomist:
- *DNR* -- Do not resuscitate. No codes should be called for this patient and no heroic measures should be taken to revive patient if the patient stops breathing.
- *NPO* -- From the Latin phrase non per os meaning nothing by mouth. Patients are not allowed food or drink including water. This restriction is usually placed on a patient before and after a procedure.
- *STAT* -- From the Latin word statim means immediately. It describes the need for a specimen or test to be done immediately in response to critical situations with the possibility of the test results preventing a patient's death.
- *ASAP* -- As soon as possible, this is used if the results are needed soon but not to prevent the patient from dying
- *Fasting* -- When a person refrains from eating or drinking anything before a procedure, sometimes water is allowed on a fast

Advising patients

The phlebotomist's responsibility is not to inform a patient of his prognosis; this is the responsibility of the patient's physician. The phlebotomist may not know all the facts of the case and may give false and detrimental information to the patient. Encourage the patient to ask the physician about the prognosis.

When asked about a collection being drawn, do not discuss in detail what is being tested for since there can be various reasons why a test was ordered by the patient's physician. Respond to the patient that the physician has ordered these test as a part of the patient's medical care and that if they have any questions about them please ask the physician.

Patient identification

Proper patient identification is important because it can prevent a critical error like misidentifying a patient specimen which could result in harm or death to a patient. Patient identification includes asking a patient to state their name and date of birth, and then you check the identification band and the requisition to see if they match. Verbal identification should never be relied on alone although it is important since patients can be hard of hearing, ill, or mentally incompetent and may give incorrect information. Also, check the identification band since it is possible for a patient o be wearing the wrong ID band. If there is no ID band, notify the nurse and have her confirm the patient's identity and attach an ID band before the blood is drawn. If there is any discrepancy on the ID band, information given by the patient or on the requisition, a reconciliation of the discrepancy must be made before a collection is taken. More than one patient may have the same name. Usually a name alert is placed on the chart but not in all cases.

Sleeping patients
Drawing blood from a sleeping patient might startle the patient and could change testing results. Also, you or the patient could be injured as the result of the patient being startled. The appropriate action to take would be to gently say the patient's name and shake the bed (never the patient) to wake them up.

Equipment selection

This allows you to waste less equipment if your collection site turns out to be inappropriate for the equipment you have assembled. Also, this allows for adequate drying time for the alcohol which allows for proper cleaning of the site and reduced sting from the alcohol. A site should have a minimum drying time of 30 seconds.

Basal state

Basal state defined -- The basal state is defined at the condition of the body early in the morning while the body is at rest and has been fasting for about 12 hours. For example a patient who at dinner at 5:00PM and wakes at 5:00AM is close to his or her body's basal state.

Factors influencing basal state -- Age, altitude, daily variations, dehydration, diet, drugs (prescription and illegal), exercise, fever, gender, humidity, jaundice, position, pregnancy, smoking, stress, and temperature

Patient issues

Many patients have allergies. These include possible allergies to adhesives, latex, and antiseptics. A patient may have a bleeding or bruising disorder that results from a genetic reason or medication that they are taking. Some patients may faint (syncope) during a procedure. It is very appropriate to recline a patient or have the lay down if they have fainted before. Some patients have a fear of needles. Some may experience nausea and vomiting from fear or an illness they have. It may be necessarily to have a trash can or spit-up container near by for easy access. If a patient his overweight or obese then it may make a collection difficult.

Site selection

Some variables that make a site inappropriate for selection:
- Injuries to the skin such as burns, scars, and tattoos
- Damaged veins from repeated collections or drug use
- Swelling (edema)
- Hematoma (bruising)
- Mastectomy or cancer removal including skin cancer

Poor phlebotomy technique

A hematoma can result from errors in phlebotomy techniques:
- Inadequate pressure to the collection site after a blood draw
- Blood leaking through the back of a vein that was pierced
- Blood leaking from a partial pierced vein
- An artery is pierced

<u>Some of the risks to patients if a complication or error results from blood collection</u>:

- Arterial puncture
- Anemia resulting from the procedure
- Infection
- Hematoma (bruising) of the venipuncture site
- Damage to a nerve if punctured
- Vein damage
- Pain

Wipe away first droplet

The first droplet of blood contains excess tissue fluid which may affect test results. Also, the alcohol residue on the skin will be wiped away with the first droplet of blood. The alcohol can hemolyze the blood specimen and keep a round droplet of blood from forming.

Retrieving blood from children

Skin puncture is the preferred method for retrieving blood from a child or infant because children have smaller quantities of blood than adults which can lead to anemia if enough blood is drawn. Also, a child or infant may be hurt if they need to be restrained during a venipuncture. Also, infants may go into cardiac arrest if more than 10% of their blood volume is removed. If a child moves around during venipuncture, it may result in an injury to nerves, veins, and arteries.

<u>Infant heel punctures</u>
NCCLS states that the safest areas for skin puncture in an infant are on the plantar surface of the hell, medial to the imaginary line extending from the middle of the big toe to the heel or lateral to an imaginary line extending from between the fourth and fifth toes to the heel. Deep punctures of an infant's heel can lead to osteochondritis (inflammation of the bone and cartilage) and osteomyelitis (inflammation of the bone).

<u>Recommended skin puncture site for older children and young adults</u>
The recommended site for skin puncture for this age group is the fleshy portion on the palmar surface of the distal segment of the middle or ring finger.

Blood smears

A blood smear will be spread over one-half to three-fourths of the slide. There will be a gradual shift from thick to thin blood smear on the slide with the thinnest part of the slide being one blood cell thick. This thinnest part of the blood smear is sometimes referred to as the "feather." The feather part of the blood smear is the most important since the differential is performed there. In blood smears made using the two slide method hold the slide that will smear the blood droplet at a 30 degree angle to the slide that the blood droplet was placed on.

Glucose tolerance tests

A patient should eat balanced meals with 150 grams of carbohydrates for 3 days the should refrain from eating 12 hours before the test as well as not smoking or chewing gum before or during the testing period.

Age and weight requirements

The donor must be between the ages of 17 and 66. The donor must weigh at least 110 lbs.

Ethics

Steps in the ethical decision making process:
- Identify the health problem.
- Define the ethical issue.
- Gather additional information.
- Delineate the decision maker.
- Examine ethical and moral principles.
- Explore alternative options.
- Implement decisions.
- Evaluate and modify actions.

Negligence and Malpractice
Negligence: and unintentional tort involving a breach of duty or failure (through an act or an omission) to meet a standard of care, causing patient harm.

Malpractice: a type of professional liability based on negligence in which the health care professional is held accountable for breach of a duty of care involving special knowledge and skill.

Arterial blood pH

7.35-7.45 is the normal range for arterial blood pH. Acidosis describes below normal blood pH. Alkalosis describes above normal blood pH.

pH is the measure of the acidity of a solution. pH is equal to the negative logarithm of the concentration of hydrogen ions in a solution. A pH of 7 is neutral. Values less than 7 are acidic, and values greater than 7 are basic. A range of 6.5 to 7.5 is considered a neutral environment.

General information

The following is important general information for the phlebotomist:
- A typical blood donor unit contains 450 mL of blood.
- A paternity test cannot prove to a complete certainty that a specific male has fathered a child. It can rule out with certainty that a man did not father a specific child.
- Sugarless foods can affect the digestive process which in turn can affect the glucose tolerance test results.
- Turnaround time starts when the order is received not when the draw of the testing specimen is completed.
- An arteriospasm can occur when proper technique is used. It is a reflexive constricting of the artery possibly caused by anxiety, pain or arterial muscle irritation.
- Arterial puncture is more painful than venipuncture, but it should not be extremely painful. Extreme pain indicates that a nerve has been involved in the procedure, and the procedure should stop.
- Vasovagal syncope is due hypotension as the result of abrupt pain or trauma.The best way to tell if a specimen is arterial is by the way the blood pumps into the syringe.
- Wrapping a specimen in alumium foil is a good way to protect it from light.
- According to NCCLS guidelines, a specimen should be separated ASAP with 2 hours being the absolute time limit.

- A cold agglutinin requires special transportation at body temperature.
- If unfamilar with a requested test, a phlebotomist should refer to the laboratory user manual for information and instructions about the test.

Potassium

Potassium is represented by the letter K. It is an electrolyte that helps maintain the body's homeostasis. The body maintains its levels of potassium in a very narrow range since too much or too little of an electrolyte can result in death if the imbalance is not corrected. The roles that potassium fills in the human body include maintain the acidic and basic balance, assisting in muscle functions, assisting with nerve conduction and maintaining osmotic pressure. Another major role that it plays involves the heart's cardiac output; it assists in this by controlling the heart rate and the heart's contraction force.

Ulnar artery

The ulnar artery provides collateral circulation for the hand. Since the radial artery is most commonly used in arterial puncture, the ulnar artery is there as a back up to provide blood to the hand if the radial artery is damaged and becomes unable to supply blood to the hand.

Arterial punctures

Some of the most common sites for arterial punctures:
- The radial artery is the preferred choice for arterial puncture. It is located on the thumb site of the wrist and is most commonly used.
- The brachial artery is second choice. It is located in the medial anterior aspect of the antecubital area near the biceps tendon insertion.
- Femoral artery is only used by physicians and trained ER personnel. It is usually used in emergency situations or with patients with low cardiac output.

Applying pressure after puncture

For 3 to 5 minutes directly after the needle is withdrawn from an arterial puncture, a phlebotomist should apply pressure to the puncture site. A patient should not be allowed to hold pressure since they may not hold adequate pressure for the required length of time.

Allen test

The purpose of the Allen's test is to determine the presence of collateral circulation in the hand by the ulnar artery.

- Compress the radial and ulnar arteries with fingers while the patient makes a fist.
- Patient opens hand; it should have a blanched appearance.
- The ulnar artery is released and the patient's hand should flush with color. If this occurs, the patient has a positive Allen test and has collateral circulation of the ulnar artery.

Locating pulse failure

If you are unable to find a pulse after an arterial puncture or the pulse is faint, blood flow may be blocked partially or completely by a blood clot. Notify the patient's nurse or physician STAT so that circulation can begin to be restored as quickly as possible.

Urine specimen collection

All urine must be collected over the course of 24 hours. A large collection container is given to the patient. When a patient awakes, the first void of the morning is for the previous 24 hours and must be discarded. The next void is collected as well as the next void over the next 24 hours as well as the next morning void. Sometimes the specimen collection has to be refrigerated.

Some common urine tests and what they are commonly used to find:

- Routine Urinalysis
- Culture and Sensitivity – diagnosis urinary tract infection
- Cytology Studies – presence of abnormal cells from urinary tract
- Drug Screening – detects illegal use of drugs (prescription or illicit) and steroid, also monitors therapeutic drug use.
- Pregnancy Test – confirms pregnancy by testing for the presence of HCG

- 55 -

Nonblood fluid specimens

- Urine
- Amniotic Fluid
- Cerebrospinal Fluid
- Gastric Secretions
- Nasopharyngeal Secretions
- Saliva
- Semen
- Serous Fluids
- Sputum
- Sweat
- Synovial Fluid

Midstream urine collection

Both midstream and clean-catch involve an initial void into the toilet, interruption of urine flow, the restart of urination into a collection container, collection of a sufficient amount of specimen, and voiding of excess urine down the toilet.

The *clean-catch* involves cleaning of the genital area, collecting urine into a sterile container and quick processing to prevent overgrowth of microorganisms, degradation of the specimen, and incorrect results.

AFP

AFP is alpha-fetoprotein. Normally it is found in the human fetus, but abnormal levels of AFP may indicate a neural tube defect in an infant or another fetal developmental problem. The test is performed on maternal serum. If results are abnormal, a test on the amniotic fluid will be used to confirm results.

Aspects reviewed routinely

The following are aspects of an analysis routinely reviewed:
- Physical- color, odor, transparency, specific gravity
- Chemical- looking for bacteria, blood, WBC, protein, and glucose
- Microscopic – urine components i.e. casts, cells, and crystals

LIS

An LIS is a laboratory information system. Usually the LIS is used to order tests, print labels for specimens, and enter test results. LIS can be customized to specific laboratory requirements.

Passwords

A password is unique to each computer user. It should be kept confidential. A password allows access to a computer and identifies who the computer user is when used in conjunction with an ID code. When the ID code or password is used to obtain access to a computer, this is called logging on.

Inverting a tube

A tube should be inverted if it contains an additive and if the manufacturer's instructions require for it to be inverted. If the tube in a nonadditive tube then it does not have to be inverted. An additive tube usually is inverted between three and eight times to properly mix the additive with the blood.

Computer-generated labels

The label would contain the patient's name, date of birth or age, medical record number, collection time (in military time).

Proper handling

46 to 68% of lab errors result from improper handling of a specimen before it was analyzed. For example, if an anticoagulant tube is improperly mixed, it may result in microclots forming. If a tube is shaken too hard hemolysis of the specimen may occur. If a specimen is not cooled properly then metabolic processes may continue after collection which may skew test results.

Most appropriate way to chill a specimen
The most appropriate way to chill a specimen is to immerse it into an ice and water slush. Ice cubes alone will not allow for adequate cooling of the specimen, and where the ice cubes touch the specimen may freeze it resulting in possible hemolysis or breakdown of the analyte.

Three types of heparin

The purpose of heparin is to prevent coagulation. The three types of heparin are ammonium, sodium and lithium. Ammonium heparin is used for hematocrit determinations and is found in capillary tubes. Sodium heparin and lithium heparin are used in evacuated tubes. Just be sure that the heparin that is being used is not what is being tested. For example heparin is used for electrolyte testing, but sodium is a commonly tested electrolyte thus sodium heparin would not be an appropriate heparin to use to test for electrolytes. It is important to mix heparin tubes properly to prevent microclots.

Aliquot

When a specimen is collected, it may need to be divided to run several test on it. An aliquot is a fraction of the specimen. Each aliquot has its own tube for testing and is label with the same information as the original specimen.

Electrolyte analysis

Bicarbonate, chloride, potassium and sodium are the four most commonly tested for electrolytes.

Proper centrifuge

The centrifuge needs to be evenly balanced with tubes of equal size and volume across from one another. Stoppers should always be in place to prevent aerosol. Also, be sure to allow complete clotting before centrifuging the specimen. If a specimen is not completely clotted before centrifuging then it may result in latent fibrin formations clotting the serum. Never centrifuge a specimen twice.

Preventing aerosol formation

The stopper should be covered with 4x4-inch gauze and placed behind a safety shield to ensure the aerosol is not inhaled. Proper protective clothing should be worn as well. A safety stopper removal device may also be used.

RAM and ROM

RAM is temporary computer data storage. RAM stands for Random Access Memory. If RAM is not saved into a permanent file the information will be lost if the computer is turned off.

ROM is read-only memory. ROM is memory whose contents can be accessed and read but cannot be easily changed. When a computer is turned off and turned back on the ROM has not changed.

How blood settles

How blood in an anticoagulant tube with settle after being centrifuged or being allowed to settle:
- The top layer will be the plasma.
- The next thin layer is the buffy coat made of white blood cells and platelets.
- The bottom layer is red blood cells.

Specimen rejection

Some reasons why a specimen may be rejected for testing include incorrect or incomplete identification, collected in an expired tube, inadequate amount of specimen collected (QNS, quantity not sufficient), and collection in an incorrect tube.

Analytes broken down

Some commonly tested for analytes that can be broken down in the presence of light:
- Bilirubin
- Vitamin B_{12}
- Urine Prophyrins

Important Terms

Blood smear -- Blood layer on a glass slide made from a drop of blood
Capillary blood gases -- Blood gases retrieved from an arterialized skin puncture
Interstitial fluid -- Liquid found between cells
Intracellular fluid -- Liquid found within cell membranes

Accession Number -- Unique number given for each test request

Aerosol -- Substance released in the form of a fine mist

Barcode -- Series of black bars and white spaces spaced at intentional, unique distances to represent numbers and letters

Centrifugation -- The process of substance separation by spinning

Impermeable -- Does not allow the passage of liquids

CPU -- Central Processing Unit, the command center of the computer

Cursor -- Blinking marker on the computer screen that indicates where information should be inputted

Hardware -- The mechanical, magnetic, electronic, and electrical components making up a computer system

Interface -- A connection between hardware devices, applications, or different sections of a computer network

Monitor -- A device similar to a television screen that receives video signals from the computer and displays the information for the user

Practice Test

Practice Questions

1. Transfer of an infectious agent via droplets larger than 5 μm in diameter is known as
    a. Airborne transmission
    b. Droplet transmission
    c. Vector transmission
    d. Vehicle transmission

2. Which of the following is an example of vector transmission?
    a. Tuberculosis
    b. Salmonella infection
    c. Bubonic plague
    d. HIV

3. Droplet transmission may result from
    a. Mosquito bite
    b. Kissing
    c. Contaminated food or water
    d. Throat swab

4. All of the following are prohibited under Centers for Disease Control (CDC) guidelines for hand hygiene **EXCEPT**
    a. Hand washing using plain soap and water
    b. Artificial nails
    c. Nails longer than one quarter inch
    d. Touching faucet handles after hand washing

5. Protective isolation may be required for all of the following patients **EXCEPT**
    a. Neutropenic chemotherapy patients
    b. Burn patients
    c. Infants
    d. AIDS patients

6. Which of the following statements regarding standard precautions for infection control is **FALSE**?

    a. Use both hands to recap needles

    b. Hands should be washed before putting on and after removing gloves

    c. Standard precautions apply to all secretions except sweat

    d. Resuscitation devices may be used as an alternative to the mouth-to-mouth method

7. Use of an N95 respirator is **NOT** required in the case of

    a. A child with chickenpox

    b. A child with measles

    c. An adult immune to measles or chickenpox

    d. An adult who has never had measles or chickenpox

8. Which of the following is **NOT** a violation of general laboratory safety rules?

    a. Wearing a laboratory coat when leaving the lab

    b. Wearing nail polish

    c. Wearing large earrings

    d. Having shoulder-length hair

9. Which of the following statements regarding HBV is **FALSE**?

    a. HBV vaccine also protects against HDV

    b. HBV vaccine does not contain live virus

    c. HBV vaccine may pose a risk of HBV transmission

    d. HBV can survive up to 1 week in dried blood

10. HCV exposure may occur through

    a. Urine

    b. Sexual contact

    c. Semen

    d. Phlebotomy procedures

11. To reduce the risk of transmission of a bloodborne pathogen, you should

    a. Cleanse the wound with bleach

    b. Cleanse the wound with an antiseptic

    c. Cleanse the wound with soap and water

    d. Squeeze the wound to release fluid

12. A specific type of fire extinguisher is used for each of the following classes of fire **EXCEPT**
    a. Class K
    b. Class D
    c. Class C
    d. Class B

13. A fire caused by the splashing of hot grease from a frying pan is classified as a
    a. Class K fire
    b. Class A fire
    c. Class B fire
    d. Class D fire

14. All of the following are acceptable procedures to control wound hemorrhage **EXCEPT**
    a. Applying direct pressure to the wound
    b. Using an elastic bandage to hold the compress
    c. Removing the original compress when adding additional material
    d. Using cloth or gauze to apply pressure

15. Which of the following symbols is **NOT** included on the Joint Commission "Do Not Use" list?
    a. IU
    b. IV
    c. U
    d. QD

16. Which symbol may soon be included in the Joint Commission "Do Not Use" list?
    a. Minus sign (-)
    b. Equal sign (=)
    c. Plus-or-minus sign (±)
    d. Less than sign (<)

17. A patient lying with his palm facing down is said to be in the
    a. Anatomic position
    b. Prone position
    c. Supine position
    d. Reclining position

18. Which of the following statements regarding lumbar puncture is **FALSE**?
    a. The needle enters the spinal cavity
    b. The needle enters the space between the 3rd and 4th lumbar vertebrae
    c. The procedure poses a risk of injury to the spinal cord
    d. The procedure does not present a risk of spinal cord injury

19. The hormone epinephrine
    a. Increases blood pressure and heart rate
    b. Controls thyroid activity
    c. Is associated with SAD
    d. Decreases urine production

20. Increased levels of which of the following are associated with heart attack?
    a. Albumin
    b. PSA
    c. CK
    d. CEA

21. The most frequent source of carryover contamination is
    a. Heparin
    b. EDTA tubes
    c. PTT
    d. Coagulation tubes

22. Which of the following is the recommended order of draw for syringes?
    a. The SST follows the red top
    b. The red top follows the SST
    c. The gray top is first
    d. Sterile specimens are last

23. According to the alternate order of draw for syringes,
   a. The light-blue top is first
   b. The lavender top is first
   c. The red top and SST are last
   d. The gray top is last

24. A sign with a picture of fall leaves may be used to indicate
   a. Do not resuscitate order
   b. Miscarriage
   c. No blood pressures in right arm
   d. Fall precautions

25. Which of the following statements regarding obtaining a blood specimen from a patient is **FALSE**?
   a. The phlebotomist should ask the patient's permission before collecting blood
   b. The patient has the right to refuse blood draw
   c. The name of the ordering physician on the ID band should not differ
   d. Patient identity should always be verified

26. Which of the following statements regarding patient identification is **FALSE?**
   a. Outpatients may be identified by an ID card
   b. Outpatients should be asked to state their name and date of birth
   c. If a patient has been identified by the receptionist, no further verification is needed
   d. A patient's response when his or her name is called is not sufficient for identification

27. The preferred venipuncture site is the
   a. Cephalic vein
   b. Median cubital vein
   c. Median basilic vein
   d. Median cephalic vein

28. All of the following statements regarding tourniquet application are true **EXCEPT**
     a. The patient should be told to pump his fist
     b. A tourniquet may be applied over the patient's sleeve
     c. Two tourniquets may be used together
     d. A tourniquet should not be applied over an open sore

29. An outpatient's blood should **NOT** be drawn
     a. While reclining in a chair
     b. While lying down
     c. Unless seated in a blood-drawing chair
     d. While seated on a stool

30. When selecting a vein for venipuncture, you should
     a. Select a vein close to a pulse
     b. Use the basilic vein as an alternative if the median cubital vein cannot be located
     c. Palpate visible veins
     d. Use your thumb to palpate a vein

31. If an antecubital vein cannot be located, you may
     a. Use a vein on the underside of the wrist
     b. Perform a capillary puncture
     c. Manipulate the site until a vein can be found
     d. Use a tendon

32. Proper technique for needle insertion includes
     a. Pushing down on the needle
     b. Using a C hold
     c. Using an L hold
     d. Advancing the needle slowly

33. Which of the following statements regarding blood specimens is **FALSE**?
     a. Outpatient and inpatient blood specimens have the same normal values
     b. Hemoglobin and hematocrit have higher normal ranges at higher elevations
     c. Caffeine may affect cortisol levels
     d. Ingestion of butter or cheese may produce a milky specimen

34. Blood levels of which of the following are normally lowest during the morning?
    a. Iron
    b. Insulin
    c. Potassium
    d. Glucose

35. Exercise increases levels of all of the following **EXCEPT**
    a. Protein
    b. Cholesterol
    c. Liver enzymes
    d. Skeletal muscle enzymes

36. All of the following affect blood specimen composition **EXCEPT**
    a. Body position
    b. Temperature and humidity
    c. Fasting
    d. Stress

37. In which of the following patients is blood collection prohibited?
    a. Patient with a hematoma
    b. Pregnant patient
    c. Mastectomy patient
    d. Patient with a tattoo

38. In a patient with an IV, blood should **NOT** be drawn
    a. By capillary puncture
    b. Below the IV
    c. Above the IV
    d. From a different vein

39. In obtaining a blood specimen in a patient with an IV, the phlebotomist should
    a. Turn off the IV
    b. Restart the IV after venipuncture
    c. Select a site proximal to the IV
    d. Apply a tourniquet distal to the IV

40. A patient begins to faint during blood collection. The most appropriate line of action would be to

    a. Use an ammonia inhalant to revive the patient

    b. Continue the draw and quickly withdraw the needle

    c. Apply pressure to the site and lower the patient's head

    d. Allow the patient to leave after regaining consciousness

41. All of the following may trigger hematoma **EXCEPT**

    a. Small veins

    b. Inadequate pressure to the site

    c. Needle penetration all the way through the vein

    d. Petechiae

42. To prevent hemoconcentration during venipuncture, you should

    a. Massage the area until a vein is located

    b. Ask the patient to release his or her fist when blood flow begins

    c. Ask the patient to vigorously pump his or her fist

    d. Redirect the needle several times until a vein is located

43. Hemolysis may result from all of the following **EXCEPT**

    a. Filling the tube until the normal amount of vacuum is exhausted

    b. Partially filling a sodium fluoride tube

    c. Liver disease

    d. Pulling back the plunger too quickly

44. Under which of the following conditions is underfilling additive tubes **UNACCEPTABLE**?

    a. When drawing blood from children

    b. When drawing blood from anemic patients

    c. When using a red top or SST

    d. As a time-saving strategy

45. Which of the following is **NOT** a cause of vein collapse?

    a. Tourniquet too close to the venipuncture site

    b. Vacuum draw of the tube

    c. Stoppage of blood flow on tourniquet removal

    d. Rolling veins

46. Capillary puncture is the preferred method for
    a. Dehydrated patients
    b. Newborns
    c. Coagulation studies
    d. Blood cultures

47. The recommended site for capillary puncture is the
    a. Tip of the finger
    b. Big toe
    c. Index finger
    d. Middle finger

48. A safe area for capillary puncture in infants is the
    a. Medial plantar surface of the heel
    b. Posterior curvature of the heel
    c. Arch of the foot
    d. Earlobe

49. Which of the following statements regarding warming techniques is **FALSE**?
    a. Warming the site is necessary for collecting blood gas specimens
    b. Warming is required for fingersticks in patients with cold hands
    c. Warming significantly alters results of routine analyte testing
    d. Warming is recommended for heelstick procedures in infants

50. Proper blood collection procedure includes
    a. Wiping away the first drop of blood
    b. Applying strong repetitive pressure on the site
    c. Using a scooping motion to collect blood as it flows down the finger
    d. Removing the tube from the drop

51. Proper procedure for capillary puncture in an infant or small child includes
    a. Grasping only the finger to be used for puncture
    b. Grasping all of the fingers at the same time
    c. Applying a bandage after specimen collection
    d. Placing the child face down

52. Proper procedure for TB testing includes
   a. Applying pressure to the site
   b. Wiping the site with gauze
   c. Avoiding areas of the arm with excessive hair
   d. Applying a bandage to the site

53. Therapeutic phlebotomy is used for all of the following **EXCEPT**
   a. Polycythemia
   b. Toxicology studies
   c. Hemochromatosis
   d. Large-volume blood withdrawal

54. Collection timing is most critical for
   a. Phenobarbital
   b. Digoxin
   c. Ethanol
   d. Aminoglycosides

55. Which of the following disinfectants may be used for ETOH testing?
   a. Tincture of iodine
   b. Soap and water
   c. Isopropyl alcohol
   d. Methanol

56. Abnormal bone function caused by a lack of vitamin D in the diet is known as
   a. Arthritis
   b. Osteochondritis
   c. Rickets
   d. Osteomyelitis

57. Which of the following is a form of arthritis?
   a. Bursitis
   b. Gout
   c. Rickets
   d. Slipped disc

58. Which of the following is used to test thyroid function?
    a. GH
    b. GTT
    c. ADH
    d. TSH

59. A type of diagnostic test used for cystitis is
    a. ACTH
    b. TSH
    c. C & S
    d. FBS

60. An individual with which type of blood can be a blood donor to individuals with any of the four blood types?
    a. Type A
    b. Type B
    c. Type AB
    d. Type O

61. An individual with which type of blood can receive all 4 blood types?
    a. Type A
    b. Type B
    c. Type AB
    d. Type O

62. The Rh factor is also known as the
    a. A antigen
    b. B antigen
    c. AB antigen
    d. D antigen

63. A condition marked by a decrease in the number of red blood cells is known as
    a. Anemia
    b. Leukemia
    c. Thrombocytopenia
    d. Polycythemia

64. The butterfly infusion set is used for all of the following types of patients **EXCEPT**
    a. Infants
    b. Obese patients
    c. Adults with small wrists
    d. Elderly patients

65. Which of the following statements regarding arterial puncture is **FALSE**?
    a. The patient should be checked for allergies before the procedure
    b. A patient afraid of needles should be calmed down
    c. A phlebotomist may be trained to perform the procedure
    d. The chance of a hematoma is increased

66. Intraoperative blood collection may be used in which type of surgery?
    a. Transplant
    b. Cancer
    c. Lower GI tract
    d. Pediatric

67. Which of the following statements regarding special blood collection procedures is **FALSE**?
    a. Blood pressure cannot be performed on an AV shunt
    b. Coagulation studies cannot be drawn from a heparin lock
    c. A heparin lock may be left in the vein for 48 hours
    d. An implanted port should be covered with a bandage

68. The proper pH level for arterial blood is
    a. 5.35-5.45
    b. 7.35-7.45
    c. 3.35-3.45
    d. 2.35-2.45

69. For blood collection with the butterfly infusion set in a child, you should use a
    a. 23-gauge needle with a 5-mL tube
    b. 21-gauge needle with a 5-mL tube
    c. 23-gauge needle with a 2-mL tube
    d. 22-gauge needle with a 2-mL tube

70. A normal hematocrit level for a newborn is
    a. 42-52%
    b. 51-61%
    c. 36-48%
    d. 34-42%

71. A patient's blood glucose level is usually elevated
    a. After fasting
    b. After ingesting a low-carbohydrate meal
    c. After ingesting a high-carbohydrate meal
    d. Two hours after ingesting a high-carbohydrate meal

72. The normal range for blood glucose level in a healthy adult is
    a. 65-110 mg/dL
    b. 45-65 mg/dL
    c. 55-75 mg/dL
    d. 45-90 mg/dL

73. All of the following are blood gas values **EXCEPT**
    a. pH
    b. BUN
    c. pCO_2
    d. Hct

74. The most plentiful electrolyte in serum or plasma is
    a. Potassium
    b. Sodium
    c. Chloride
    d. Calcium

75. Both sodium and potassium play a major role in
    a. Osmotic pressure
    b. Muscle function
    c. Cardiac output
    d. Renal function

76. Which of the following statements regarding HCG testing is **FALSE**?

    a. Contaminants such as detergent may invalidate results

    b. Medications may produce false-negative results

    c. Positive results are available the first week after conception

    d. Ovarian tumors may increase levels

77. Which of the following characteristics of a urine sample is indicative of a pathological condition?

    a. White or pigmented yellow foam

    b. Dark amber color

    c. Epithelial cells

    d. Bacteria

78. A urine sample is considered acidic at a pH of

    a. 7

    b. Less than 7

    c. Greater than 7

    d. 3

79. All of the following are indicative of a UTI **EXCEPT**

    a. Leukocytes

    b. Nitrites

    c. Protein

    d. Glucose

80. Trough levels are collected

    a. 30 to 60 minutes after the drug is administered

    b. To screen for drug intoxication

    c. Prior to administration of the next dose

    d. For DNA testing

81. TB is diagnosed using the

    a. Schick test

    b. PPD test

    c. Dick test

    d. Histo test

82. All of the following cannot be ingested prior to a fecal occult blood test **EXCEPT**
    a. Vitamin C
    b. Aspirin
    c. Spinach
    d. Horseradish

83. Which of the following is **NOT** normally present in the urine?
    a. Ketones
    b. Bilirubin
    c. Albumin
    d. Bacteria

84. Which of the following specimens must be kept at or near body temperature?
    a. Lactic acid
    b. Ammonia
    c. Glucagon
    d. Cryoglobulin

85. The ___ plane divides the body into top and bottom halves.
    a. Sagittal
    b. Midsagittal
    c. Transverse
    d. Frontal

86. The abbreviation Q2H indicates that the drug should be given
    a. Twice a day
    b. Every hour
    c. By mouth
    d. Every 2 hours

87. The most common type of tissue found in the body is
    a. Connective
    b. Muscle
    c. Epithelial
    d. Nerve

88. The total number of bones in the body is
    a. 200
    b. 100
    c. 206
    d. 106

89. The total number of muscles in the body is
    a. 566
    b. 656
    c. 556
    d. 560

90. The area between neurons over which impulses jump is known as the
    a. Axon
    b. Dendrite
    c. Synapse
    d. Myelin sheath

91. The gray matter of the brain is composed of
    a. Myelin sheath
    b. Nonmyelinated axons
    c. Schwann cells
    d. Synapses

92. The PNS is composed of
    a. Cranial nerves
    b. Optic nerves
    c. Spinal cord
    d. CNS

93. Hydrocephalus is characterized by
    a. Stiff neck
    b. Nerve pain
    c. Shuffling gait
    d. Enlarged head

94. The outermost layer of the skin is known as the
    a. Dermis
    b. Epidermis
    c. Subcutaneous layer
    d. Hypodermal layer

95. A condition characterized by protrusion of the stomach is known as
    a. Gastritis
    b. GERD
    c. Hiatal hernia
    d. Peptic ulcer

96. The ___is a type of exocrine gland.
    a. Pancreas
    b. Pituitary
    c. Thyroid
    d. Sweat gland

97. Which of the following conditions is caused by dysfunction of the pituitary gland?
    a. Cushing syndrome
    b. Dwarfism
    c. Diabetes
    d. Parkinson disease

98. The throat is also known as the
    a. Trachea
    b. Larynx
    c. Pharynx
    d. Epiglottis

99. Asthma is caused by
    a. Obstruction of the airway
    b. Inflammation of the bronchial tubes
    c. Too rapid breathing
    d. Oxygen deficiency

100. The major portion of the heart is known as
    a. Endocardium
    b. Pericardium
    c. Myocardium
    d. Atrium

101. The pumping chambers of the heart are known as the
    a. Ventricles
    b. Atria
    c. Endocardium
    d. Septum

102. The human body has an average of __ pints of blood.
    a. 4-5
    b. 10-12
    c. 8-10
    d. 6-8

103. Approximately 92% of plasma is composed of
    a. Fibrinogen
    b. Solutes
    c. Electrolytes
    d. Water

104. A typical diagnostic test for cardiovascular disease is
    a. CBC
    b. Hgb
    c. AST
    d. ESR

105. The site typically used for testing ABGs is the
    a. Venous puncture
    b. Arterial puncture
    c. Antecubital vein
    d. Median cubital vein

106. Which type of urine specimen collection method is used in small children?
    a. Clean catch
    b. Midstream clean catch
    c. Suprapubic
    d. Regular void

107. All of the following may be used to test the CSF **EXCEPT**
    a. Chloride
    b. Total protein
    c. Glucose
    d. ABO

108. This specimen is collected 2 hours after the patient has ingested a meal
    a. FBS
    b. PP
    c. Hgb
    d. HBV

109. All of the following can affect GTT results **EXCEPT**
    a. Aspirin
    b. Birth control pills
    c. Corticosteroids
    d. Blood pressure medications

110. Which of the following is **NOT** used for coagulation monitoring?
    a. ACT
    b. Hgb
    c. PT
    d. PTT

111. Which of the following tests may be performed together to assess clotting abnormalities?
    a. ACT and PT
    b. ACT and APPT
    c. PT and PTT
    d. PT and PP

112. Which of the following statements regarding the APPT test is **FALSE**?
    a. Plasma values of 24 to 34 seconds are considered normal
    b. Whole blood values are the same as plasma values
    c. Whole blood values between 93 and 127 seconds are considered normal
    d. Plasma values differ from whole blood values

113. Which of the following tests is typically ordered stat?
    a. pCO_2
    b. HCG
    c. FBS
    d. Hgb

114. Enteric isolation procedures are required for
    a. Patients with tuberculosis
    b. Burn patients
    c. Patients with intestinal infections
    d. Patients with skin infections

115. OSHA requires that a HEPA respirator be used for
    a. Enteric isolation
    b. Burn patients
    c. Contact isolation
    d. AFB patients

116. SDS is required by OSHA for
    a. Bloodborne pathogens
    b. Electrical hazards
    c. Hazardous chemicals
    d. Radioactive hazards

117. Which of the following is **NOT** part of standard safety procedure?
    a. Recapping contaminated needles
    b. Replacing bed rails after specimen collection
    c. Reporting items dropped on the floor
    d. Reporting unusual odors

118. All of the following are required for pathogen growth **EXCEPT**
    a. Water
    b. Proper pH
    c. Heat
    d. Darkness

119. Postexposure treatment is recommended for
    a. HCV
    b. HBV
    c. HIV
    d. HBIG

120. Which of the following statements regarding HIV is **FALSE**?
    a. HIV may be transmitted through breast milk
    b. No vaccine is available for HIV
    c. Postexposure treatment is recommended for occupational exposures
    d. Those exposed to HIV must be retested 6 months after exposure

121. The source of transmission of a pathogen to others is known as the
    a. Susceptible host
    b. Reservoir host
    c. Direct contact
    d. Chain of infection

122. PPE is **NOT** required when entering the room of a patient with
    a. Skin infection
    b. Tuberculosis
    c. Intestinal infection
    d. HIV

123. Which of the following statements regarding laboratory hazards is **FALSE**?
    a. Lead aprons should be worn as a precaution for radioactive hazards
    b. Mixing bleach and ammonia creates a chemical hazard
    c. All chemical exposures require flushing the eyes or affected parts with water
    d. Electrical hazards should be removed using a broom handle

124. Which of the following information is **NOT** required on specimen tube labels?

a. Accession number

b. Physician's signature

c. Phlebotomist's initials

d. Time of test

125. All of the following are used to send laboratory requisition forms to the lab **EXCEPT**

a. Courier

b. Pneumatic tubes

c. E-mail

d. Verbal laboratory request

126. Which of the following statements regarding health care communication is **FALSE**?

a. Comfort zones are dependent on culture

b. Callers should not be put on hold

c. Sign language may be used for hearing-impaired patients

d. Sign language may be used for non–English-speaking patients

127. Which of the following constitutes negligence?

a. Intent to harm

b. Invasion of privacy

c. Injury

d. Abandonment

128. An example of an intentional tort is

a. Abandonment

b. Negligence

c. Malpractice

d. Chain of custody

129. Pre- and post- are examples of

a. Abbreviations

b. Suffixes

c. Prefixes

d. Root words

130. The term caudal means
    a. Toward the midline
    b. Toward the side
    c. Toward the head
    d. Toward the tail

131. Which of the following is **NOT** required for drug or alcohol testing?
    a. Patient consent
    b. Split sample
    c. Plastic tube
    d. Proctor

132. Bleeding time may be decreased by
    a. Blood pressure
    b. Aspirin
    c. Ethanol
    d. Dextran

133. The ACT test is used to monitor
    a. PO_2
    b. Heparin
    c. Ionized calcium
    d. Glucose

134. All of the following are trace elements **EXCEPT**
    a. Arsenic
    b. Zinc
    c. Iron
    d. Magnesium

135. Troponin is used in the diagnosis of
    a. Diabetes
    b. Heart attack
    c. Anemia
    d. Colon cancer

136. All of the following are skin tests **EXCEPT**
    a. PPD
    b. Histo
    c. BNP
    d. Cocci

137. In administering a TB test,
    a. The antigen must be injected into a vein
    b. The antigen must be injected just below the skin
    c. The degree of erythema is measured to determine a reaction
    d. Presence of a bleb or wheal indicates the antigen was injected improperly

138. A positive reaction to a TB test is indicated by
    a. Induration between 5 and 9 mm in diameter
    b. Induration less than 5 mm in diameter
    c. Induration greater than 10 mm in diameter
    d. Degree of erythema

139. All of the following are included in the procedure for strep testing **EXCEPT**
    a. Latex agglutination
    b. Nitrous acid extraction
    c. Enzyme immunoassay
    d. Specific gravity

140. Which of the following statements regarding arterial puncture is **FALSE**?
    a. Arterial puncture is more difficult to perform than venipuncture
    b. Arterial puncture is used to evaluate ABGs
    c. Arterial puncture is used for routine blood tests
    d. Arterial puncture is more painful than venipuncture

141. Decreased levels in the blood, as measured by one of the following, increase the respiration rate.
    a. PCO_2
    b. PO_2
    c. HCO_3
    d. pH

142. Base excess or deficit is calculated based on all of the following **EXCEPT**
   a. PCO_2
   b. HCO_3
   c. Hct
   d. O_2 saturation

143. Which of the following statements regarding the radial artery is **FALSE**?
   a. The radial artery may be difficult to locate in patients with low cardiac output
   b. If the radial artery is damaged, the ulnar artery may be used for arterial puncture
   c. The radial artery should not be punctured in the absence of collateral circulation
   d. The radial artery carries a higher risk of hematoma

144. The femoral artery is located in the
   a. Groin
   b. Scalp
   c. Arm
   d. Umbilical cord

145. In performing the Allen test,
   a. The patient should hyperextend the fingers
   b. Blanching of the hand indicates a positive result
   c. Both the radial and ulnar arteries should be compressed at the same time
   d. Only the radial artery should be compressed

146. In infants, which of the following sites may be used for arterial puncture?
   a. Brachial artery
   b. Umbilical artery
   c. Femoral artery
   d. Ulnar artery

147. The presence of a wheal indicates
   a. Proper injection of a local anesthetic
   b. Positive TB test
   c. Positive Allen test
   d. Improper injection of the TB antigen

148. The vasovagal response is commonly known as
    a. Allergic reaction
    b. Myocardial infarction
    c. Fainting
    d. Hematoma

149. Serous fluid may be obtained from all of the following **EXCEPT** the
    a. Peritoneal cavity
    b. Pleural cavity
    c. Pericardial cavity
    d. Spinal cavity

150. The C-urea breath test is used to detect
    a. Lactose intolerance
    b. *H pylori*
    c. Trace metals
    d. Blood disorders

Answers to Practice Questions

1. B: Droplet transmission involves transfer of an infectious agent via droplets larger than 5 μm in diameter, whereas airborne transmission involves dispersal of infectious evaporated droplet nuclei less than 5 μm in diameter. In vector transmission, infectious agents are carried by insects, arthropods, or animals; in vehicle transmission, infectious agents are transmitted through contaminated food, water, or drugs.

2. C: The transmission of bubonic plague by fleas from rodents is an example of vector transmission; tuberculosis is spread via airborne transmission. Transmission of salmonella infection associated with handling contaminated food and human immunodeficiency virus (HIV) infection through blood transfusion are examples of vehicle transmission.

3. D: Droplet transmission may result from transfer of infectious agents by coughing, sneezing, or talking or through procedures such as throat swab collection. Vector transmission may result from mosquito or flea bites and vehicle transmission though contaminated food or water; transfer of an infectious agent through kissing or touching is known as direct contact transmission.

4. A: Routine hand washing using plain soap and water is required to prevent spread of infection; alcohol-based antiseptic hand cleaners may also be used. Artificial nails or nails longer than one quarter inch are prohibited. After hand washing, a clean paper towel should be used to turn off the faucet to prevent contamination.

5. C: Protective or reverse isolation may be required for patients highly susceptible to infection, such as burn patients, patients with AIDS, or chemotherapy patients with a low neutrophil count; protective isolation is usually not required for infants.

6. A: Never use both hands to recap a needle; hands should be washed both before putting on and after removing gloves. Standard precautions should be followed for all body fluids except sweat; resuscitation devices may be used as an alternative to mouth-to-mouth resuscitation.

7. C: An N95 respirator must be worn by all individuals susceptible to measles or chickenpox before entering the room of a patient known or suspected to have these diseases; however, adults who are immune to measles or chickenpox are not required to wear an N95 respirator or surgical mask.

8. D: Shoulder-length or longer hair is acceptable in the laboratory if it is tied back; wearing nail polish or large or dangling earrings is not acceptable. A laboratory coat should never be worn when leaving the lab for any reason.

9. C: HBV vaccine does not contain live virus and thus does not carry the risk of HBV infection; HBV vaccine also protects against hepatitis D virus (HDV) because it is only contracted concurrently with HBV. HBV can survive up to 1 week in dried blood on work surfaces or other objects.

10. B: Hepatitis C virus (HCV) infection may occur through exposure to blood and serum and is primarily transmitted through sexual contact and needle sharing; however, it is rarely found in urine or semen and is not associated with phlebotomy procedures.

11. C: Cleansing the wound with plain soap and water for at least 30 seconds is useful in reducing the risk of transmission of a bloodborne pathogen; squeezing the wound or cleansing the wound with an antiseptic, bleach, or other caustic agents is not recommended.

12. B: A specific class of fire extinguisher is used for each class of fire except for class D fires; these types of fires involve combustible or reactive metals such as sodium, potassium, magnesium, or lithium and should be handled by trained firefighting personnel.

13. A: Class K fires are often caused by high-temperature cooking oils, grease, or fats; class A fires occur with wood, paper, or clothing and class B fires with flammable liquids and vapors such as paint or gasoline. Class D fires are associated with combustible or reactive materials such as sodium or potassium.

14. C: When adding additional compresses to a wound, the original compress should not be removed to avoid interference with the clotting process; direct pressure should be applied to the wound using cloth or gauze. An elastic bandage can be used to hold the compress in place.

15. B: IV is an acceptable acronym; however, IU, or international unit, is often confused with IV and thus should not be used. U should be written out as "unit" and QD as "daily."

16. D: The symbols for less than (<) and greater than (>) are often confused for the letter "L" and the number 7, respectively, and thus may soon be added to the "Do Not Use" list.

17. B: A patient lying face down or with his palm facing down is in the prone position; a patient lying on his back with his face up is in the supine position. A patient standing erect with arms at his sides and palms facing forward is in the anatomic position.

18. C: Because the spinal cord ends at the first lumbar vertebra, lumbar puncture does not present a risk of spinal cord injury. The physician inserts the needle into the spinal cavity at the space between the 3rd and 4th lumbar vertebrae.

19. A: The hormone epinephrine increases heart rate, blood pressure, and metabolic rate; the antidiuretic hormone (ADH) decreases urine production and calcitonin lowers blood calcium levels. Melatonin helps set diurnal rhythms and is associated with seasonal affective disorder (SAD).

20. C: Increased levels of creatine kinase (CK) are associated with heart attack; PSA, or prostate specific antigen, level is used to test for prostate cancer. Carcinoembryonic antigen (CEA) is used in digestive system testing and albumin in urinary system testing.

21. B: EDTA tubes are more frequently associated with carryover contamination than any other types of additives, while heparin is associated with the least amount of interference. Coagulation tubes are the first to be used because all other additive tubes interfere with coagulation tests; partial thromboplastin time (PTT) tests are affected by tissue thromboplastin contamination.

22. A: In the recommended order of draw for syringes, sterile specimens are first, followed by light-blue tops; the SST follows the red top and the gray-top tube is last.

23. C: According to the alternate syringe order of draw, the sterile specimens remain first, while the red top and SST tubes are last.

24. D: A sign with a picture of falling leaves indicates that fall precautions are required for the patient. The letters DNR indicate a do not resuscitate order, and a sign depicting a delete symbol over an arm with a needlestick indicates no blood pressures in right arm.

25. C: Occasionally, the name of the ordering physician, room number, or bed number on the patient's ID band may differ; however, patient identity must always be verified before collecting blood. As part of informed consent, patients have the right to refuse blood draw; thus, the phlebotomist must ask the patient's permission before collecting blood.

26. C: The phlebotomist should always verify a patient's ID, even if he or she has been identified by the receptionist or has responded when his or her name has been called. Some outpatients may have been issued an ID card by the clinic; however, outpatients should still be asked to confirm their name and date of birth.

27. B: Because the median cubital vein is closer to the surface and located in an area least prone to nerve damage, it is the preferred site for venipuncture. The cephalic and median cephalic veins are the second choice; the basilic and median basilic veins are least preferred because of their proximity to the median nerve and brachial artery.

28. A: When applying a tourniquet, fist pumping should be discouraged, as it may make vein location more difficult or cause changes in blood components that may affect test results. A tourniquet may be applied over a patient's sleeve if the sleeve is too tight and cannot be rolled up far enough; a tourniquet should never be placed over an open sore. Because a tourniquet may have a tendency to roll or twist on the arm of an obese patient, two tourniquets may be placed on top of each other and used together.

29. D: Blood drawing should not be performed on an outpatient who is standing or seated on a high or backless stool because of the possibility of fainting. Outpatients should be seated on a special blood-drawing chair or on a chair with armrests; however, if the patient has a tendency to faint, he or she may be seated in a reclining chair or lying down.

30. C: In selecting a vein for venipuncture, even visible veins should be palpated to judge suitability for venipuncture. If the median cubital vein cannot be located, the basilic vein should not be used unless no other vein is more prominent because of the possibility of nerve injury or damage to the brachial artery. Do not use veins that overlie or are located close to a pulse to avoid the risk of puncturing an artery. The thumb should not be used because it has a pulse and may cause a vein to be mistaken for an artery.

31. B: If an antecubital vein cannot be found on either arm, a capillary puncture may be considered provided the test can be performed on capillary blood. Veins on the underside of the wrist should not be used to avoid nerve injury; tendons should not be used as they are difficult to penetrate and lack resilience. Manipulating the site may change blood composition, which may interfere with test results.

32. C: The proper technique for anchoring the vein before venipuncture is known as the L hold technique, which involves using the fingers to support the back of the patient's arm below the elbow and placing the thumb 1 to 2 inches and slightly to the side of the venipuncture site to pull the patient's skin toward the wrist; the C hold technique, or the two-finger technique, should not be used as it may result in the needle springing back into the phlebotomist's index finger if the patient pulls his or her arm back. Pushing down on the needle during insertion is painful and may increase the risk of blood leakage; advancing the needle too slowly may prolong the patient's discomfort.

33. A: Because outpatient specimens are not obtained during the basal state, normal values may differ slightly from those of inpatients; hemoglobin (Hgb), hematocrit (Hct), and red blood cell (RBC) counts may have higher normal ranges at higher elevations. Caffeinated beverages may affect cortisol levels; ingestion of lipids such as butter or cheese may increase blood lipid content, giving blood specimens a cloudy or milky appearance.

34. D: Blood glucose levels are usually lowest in the morning; however, iron, insulin, and potassium levels are usually highest in the morning.

35. C: Exercise may increase levels of protein, insulin, glucose, and cholesterol, as well as skeletal muscle enzyme levels, but does not affect liver enzyme levels.

36. C: Body position, environmental conditions such as temperature and humidity, and stress can affect blood specimen composition; fasting is useful in eliminating dietary influences on blood testing.

37. A: Venipuncture should never be performed through a hematoma; if there is no alternative, an area distal to the hematoma should be used. In patients with a tattoo, it is best to choose another site; however, if there is no alternative, the needle should be inserted in an area that does not contain dye. In a mastectomy patient, blood should not be drawn from the arm on the same side of the mastectomy, but can be drawn from the other arm. Pregnancy does not preclude blood collection.

38. C: In a patient with an IV, blood should never be drawn from a site above the IV, as the specimen may become contaminated with IV fluid, causing erroneous test results. Venipuncture can be performed at a site distal to the IV, in a different vein than the one with the IV, or by capillary puncture.

39. D: A phlebotomist is not qualified to start or adjust an IV; rather, he or she should ask the nurse to turn off the IV at least 2 minutes before blood collection and restart the IV after venipuncture. A site distal to the IV should always be selected for venipuncture.

40. C: If a patient faints during blood collection, discontinue the draw and discard the needle; pressure should be applied to the site to prevent bleeding and bruising and the patient should be asked to lower his or her head and breathe deeply to allow oxygenated blood to access the brain. Ammonia inhalants may produce side effects such as respiratory distress in asthmatic patients and should not be used. After he or she regains consciousness, the patient should remain in the room for at least 15 minutes.

41. D: Petechiae, or small red spots that appear on the patient's skin when the tourniquet is applied, are usually caused by capillary wall defects or platelet abnormalities and are indicative of heavy bleeding at the venipuncture site; however, they are not indicative of hematoma. Using veins that are too small or fragile for the size of the needle, applying inadequate pressure to the site, and allowing the needle to penetrate all the way through the vein may cause hematoma formation.

42. B: To prevent hemoconcentration during venipuncture, the phlebotomist should ask the patient to release his or her fist when blood begins to flow; fist pumping may increase blood potassium levels and should not be encouraged. Excessively massaging the site or probing or redirecting the needle multiple times may result in hemoconcentration.

43. A: Evacuated tube system (ETS) tubes should always be filled until the normal amount of vacuum is exhausted; partially filling a normal draw sodium fluoride tube or pulling back the plunger on a syringe too quickly may result in hemolysis. Although procedural errors are the most common cause, patient conditions such as liver disease or hemolytic anemia may result in hemolysis.

44. D: Underfilling additive tubes is unacceptable as a time-saving device; underfilling is acceptable when obtaining larger amounts of blood is inadvisable, such as when drawing blood from infants or children or from severely anemic patients. Short draw serum tubes such as red tops and serum separator tubes (SSTs) are acceptable provided the specimen is not hemolyzed and there is enough of the specimen for testing.

45. C: A collapsed vein may result from the vacuum draw of the tube or pressure from pulling on the syringe or if the tourniquet is too tight or too close to the venipuncture site. Stoppage of blood flow when the tourniquet is removed may simply indicate that the needle is not positioned properly; slightly adjusting the needle usually reestablishes blood flow. Improper needle position may result in rolling veins.

46. B: Capillary puncture is the preferred method for infants and young children due to their smaller blood volume and risk of injury or serious adverse events such as anemia or cardiac arrest and is typically used for newborn screening; however, it is not appropriate for dehydrated patients or those with poor circulation. Capillary puncture cannot be used for coagulation studies, blood cultures, or tests requiring large volumes of serum or plasma.

47. D: The middle or ring finger is the recommended site for capillary puncture; the tip of the finger should not be used due to the short distance between the skin surface and bone nor the index finger because of its increased sensitivity and more frequent use. The big toe is no longer recommended as a site for capillary collection.

48. A: The medial or lateral plantar surface of the heel is the preferred site for capillary puncture; the earlobe or arch or other areas of the foot should not be used for puncture. The posterior curvature of the heel should not be used, as the bone may be only 1 mm deep in this area.

49. C: Warming of the injection site does not significantly affect results of routinely tested analytes; warming is preferred for heelstick procedures in infants due to their high red blood cell counts and is required for collection of blood gas or capillary pH specimens. Warming may be required before fingersticks in patients with cold hands.

50. A: During blood collection, the first drop of blood should be wiped away, as it may be contaminated with tissue fluid or may contain alcohol residue that may hemolyze the specimen or prevent blood from forming a well-rounded drop. Using strong repetitive pressure to milk the site may result in hemolysis or tissue fluid contamination; using a scooping motion against the skin surface may cause platelet clumping or hemolysis. Removing the tube from the site may create air spaces in the specimen that interfere with test results.

51. B: In performing a capillary puncture in an infant or small child, grasp all of the child's fingers between your fingers and thumb; grasping only one finger may cause the finger to twist if the child tries to pulls away. Bandages should not be applied to infants or children younger than 2 years of age as they may present a choking hazard or may stick and cause the skin to tear during removal. For heelstick procedures, the infant or child should be lying face up with the foot lower than the torso.

52. C: When administering a tuberculosis (TB) skin test, avoid areas of the arm with scars, bruises, burns, or excessive hair because they may interfere with test results. Applying pressure to the site may force the antigen out of the site and wiping the site with gauze may cause the antigen to be absorbed. Applying a bandage to the site may result in fluid absorption or irritation and may affect test results.

53. B: Therapeutic phlebotomy is the withdrawal of large volumes of blood and may be used as treatment for certain conditions such as polycythemia or hemochromatosis; it is not used for toxicology, or the study of toxins or poisons.

54. D: Collection timing is most critical for drugs with short half-lives, such as the aminoglycosides; timing is less critical for drugs with longer half-lives such as phenobarbital or digoxin. Timing is not essential for ethanol or blood alcohol testing.

55. B: During blood alcohol (ethanol) [ETOH] testing, regular soap and water may be used to clean the venipuncture site if an alternative disinfectant such as povidone-iodine or aqueous benzalkonium chloride is not available; disinfectants that contain alcohol such as tincture of iodine, isopropyl alcohol, or methanol should not be used, as they may compromise test results.

56. C: Rickets usually occurs in children and is marked by abnormal or "soft" bones caused by a lack of vitamin D in the diet; arthritis is an inflammatory condition of the joints. Osteochondritis is an inflammation of the bone and cartilage, and osteomyelitis is inflammation of the bone or bone marrow caused by bacterial infection.

57. B: Gout is a form of arthritis affecting the joints of the feet caused by increased uric acid levels in the blood; bursitis is an inflammation of the bursa between the muscle attachments and bone. Rickets is a condition in children caused by lack of vitamin D marked by softening and malformation of the bones; a slipped disc is a condition in which the disc between the vertebrae of the spine ruptures or protrudes out of place.

58. D: The thyroid-stimulating hormone (TSH) test is used to assess thyroid function; GH stands for growth hormone, and ADH stands for antidiuretic hormone. GTT is the glucose tolerance test.

59. C: The urine culture and sensitivity (C & S) test is used to diagnose cystitis; ACTH is used to assess adrenocorticotropic hormone and thyroid-stimulating hormone (TSH) levels. FBS is the fasting blood sugar test.

60. D: Because type O blood lacks antigens, an individual with type O blood can be a donor to individuals with any of the four blood types; thus, type O blood is known as the universal donor.

61. C: Because type AB blood lacks antibodies in its plasma, an individual with this blood type can receive blood from all 4 blood types; thus, type AB blood is known as the universal recipient.

62. D: The Rh factor is also known as the D antigen.

63. A: Anemia is a condition indicated by a deficiency of red blood cells and hemoglobin in the blood; leukemia is a condition characterized by an increase in the number of white blood cells. Thrombocytopenia is marked by a decrease in the number of platelets and polycythemia an excessive number of red blood cells.

64. B: The butterfly infusion set is used for patients with small, fragile veins, such as the elderly, infants or small children, or adults with small antecubital wrists; it is not used in obese patients.

65. C: Only physicians or specially trained emergency room personnel are qualified to perform arterial puncture; the phlebotomist is not trained to perform this procedure. Patients should be checked for allergies and must be in a steady state; thus, a patient who is afraid of needles must be calmed down before the procedure. The risk of hematoma is increased with arterial puncture.

66. A: Intraoperative blood collection is used for procedures in which the estimated amount of blood loss is 20% or more of the patient's blood volume; it is typically used in patients undergoing cardiac, vascular, gynecologic, trauma, or transplant surgery. Intraoperative blood collection is not used for cancer or lower GI tract surgery or for infants or small children due to the risk of anemia or cardiac arrest.

67. D: An implanted port is attached to an indwelling line and should not be covered with a bandage. A heparin lock is a special type of cannula that can be left in the patient's vein for up to 48 hours; however, coagulation studies should not be drawn from a heparin lock. Arteriovenous (AV) shunts are usually created to provide access for dialysis; venipuncture or blood pressure should not be performed on an AV shunt.

68. B: The pH for arterial blood should be maintained at a level of 7.35 to 7.45.

69. C: For a pediatric patient, a 23-gauge needle with a 2-mL tube should be used for butterfly infusion; use of a 5-mL tube with a 23-gauge needle may cause vein collapse or hemolysis of the specimen.

70. B: The normal hematocrit (Hct) for a newborn is within the range of 51% to 61%. For a male adult, the range should be 42% to 52%, for a female adult, 36% to 48%, and for a 6-year-old child, 34% to 42%.

71. C: A patient's blood glucose level is normally elevated after ingestion of a high-carbohydrate meal; however, glucose levels return to normal within 2 hours after ingestion.

72. A: Normal blood glucose levels for a healthy adult should range from 65 to 110 mg/dL.

73. D: Although values for hematocrit (Hct) are measured through a chemistry panel, Hct is not a blood gas value; pH, blood urea nitrogen (BUN), and partial pressure of carbon dioxide (pCO_2) are all blood gas values.

74. B: Sodium is the most plentiful electrolyte in serum or plasma.

75. A: Both sodium and potassium play a role in maintaining osmotic pressure and acid-base balance; potassium is important in maintaining muscle function and cardiac output. Blood urea nitrogen (BUN) is used to measure renal function.

76. C: Human chorionic gonadotropin (HCG) levels are increased during pregnancy; however, HCG may not be present in sufficient levels the first week or 2 after conception, and thus may yield false-negative results. Contaminants such as detergents, protein, hematuria, and bacteria as well as certain medications may invalidate results. Malignant ovarian tumors and other conditions may increase HCG levels.

77. A: A long-lasting white foam may indicate renal disease; deeply pigmented yellow foam on yellow-brown or -green urine may indicate the presence of bilirubin or biliverdin, which are associated with hepatitis. Normal urine may range in color from yellow to dark amber. Bacteria and epithelial cells are indicative of a pathological condition only when present in large quantities.

78. B: Urinary pH ranges from 5 to 9, with 7 considered neutral. Urine is considered acidic at a pH of less than 7 and alkaline at a pH of greater than 7.

79. D: A positive nitrite test in conjunction with a positive leukocyte test is indicative of urinary tract infection (UTI); a urine culture positive for blood or protein is also indicative of UTI. Glucose in the urine may be indicative of diabetes mellitus.

80. C: Trough levels are collected when the serum concentration of the drug is at its lowest level, usually just prior to administration of the next dose; peak levels are collected when the serum concentration is highest, usually 30 to 60 minutes after drug administration, and are used to screen for drug intoxication. Neither peak nor trough levels are useful for DNA testing.

81. B: The purified protein derivative (PPD) skin test is used to diagnose tuberculosis (TB); the Schick test is used in the diagnosis of diphtheria and the Dick test in the diagnosis of scarlet fever. The histoplasmosis (histo) test is used to test for infection with the organism *Histoplasmosis capsulatum*.

82. C: Prior to a fecal occult blood test, patients are prohibited from ingesting foods such as red meat, turnips, horseradish, vitamin C, aspirin, or anti-inflammatory drugs; however, patient are encouraged to eat fruits such as prunes, grapes, or apples and vegetables such as spinach, lettuce, and corn.

83. B: Bilirubin is normally present in the blood but not in the urine and is indicative of liver or gallbladder disease or cancer. Albumin is the primary protein found in urine; ketones are end products of fat metabolism and normally present in the urine. Bacteria may be present in the urine in small amounts; only large quantities of bacteria are indicative of pathology.

84. D: Cryoglobulin, cryofibrinogen, and cold agglutinin specimens must be kept at or near body temperature; lactic acid, ammonia, and glucagon specimens require chilling.

85. C: The transverse plane divides the body into top and bottom halves; the sagittal plane divides the body into unequal right and left halves and the midsagittal plane into equal right and left halves. The frontal plane is parallel to the long axis of the body and at right angles to the midsagittal plane.

86. D: The abbreviation q stands for "every"; thus, Q2H means that the drug should be given every 2 hours. BID indicates that the drug should be administered twice a day and PO means given orally (from the Latin *per os*), or by mouth.

87. A: Connective tissue is the most common type of tissue found in the body; muscle tissue is essential for movement and epithelial tissue protects the internal and external structures of the body. Nerve tissue consists of cells that send and receive information.

88. C: There are a total of 206 bones in the human body.

89. B: There are a total of 656 muscles in the body.

90. C: The synapse is the area between neurons over which impulses literally jump to transmit messages; dendrites and axons are extensions of the neuron. The myelin sheath covers the axon and increases the speed of a nerve impulse.

91. B: The white matter of the brain is composed of the myelin sheath; nonmyelinated axons are not covered by the myelin sheath and are known as the gray matter. Schwann cells are a fatty substance that composes the myelin sheath; synapses are areas between neurons over which impulses jump to transmit messages.

92. A: The peripheral nervous system (PNS) is located outside of the central nervous system (CNS) and is composed of the cranial nerves except the optic nerve, the spinal nerves, and the autonomic nervous system. The spinal cord and brain compose the CNS.

93. D: Hydrocephalus is an increased volume of cerebrospinal fluid in the brain at birth and is characterized by an enlargement of the infant's head; headache, stiff neck, and fever are symptoms of meningitis, or an inflammation of the meninges of the brain. A shuffling gait, muscular rigidity, and tremor are characteristic of Parkinson disease, and nerve pain is characteristic of neuralgia.

94. B: The outermost layer of the skin is known as the epidermis; the second layer, or the dermis, is thicker than the epidermis and is known as the "true skin." The subcutaneous or hypodermal layer lies underneath the dermis.

95. C: Hiatal hernia is a condition marked by protrusion of the stomach through a weak area of the diaphragm; gastritis is an acute or chronic inflammation of the stomach lining, and peptic ulcer is erosion of the stomach lining. Gastroesophageal reflux disease (GERD) is a relaxation of the lower sphincter muscle that allows the contents of the stomach to move up the esophagus.

96. D: Sweat glands are a type of exocrine gland, which is composed of ducts that carry secretions to the body surface or to organs. The pancreas, pituitary, and thyroid are endocrine glands, or ductless glands that secrete hormones directly into the bloodstream.

97. B: Dwarfism is caused by hypofunctioning of the pituitary gland in childhood; Cushing syndrome is caused by hypersecretion of the glucocorticoid hormone and diabetes by reduced secretion of insulin from the pancreas. Parkinson disease is a disorder of the peripheral nervous system.

98. C: The throat is also known as the pharynx; the larynx is known as the voice box, and the trachea is known as the windpipe. The epiglottis is a covering of the opening of the larynx that causes food to pass down the esophagus rather than the trachea.

99. A: Asthma is caused by obstruction of the airway due to inflammation; bronchitis is caused by inflammation of the bronchial tubes. Hyperventilation is characterized by rapid breathing resulting in a loss of carbon dioxide. Hypoxia is caused by oxygen deficiency.

100. C: The major portion of the heart is known as the myocardium; the pericardium is a layer of fibrous tissue that surrounds the heart, and the endocardium covers the inner layer of the heart. The atrium is the receiving chamber of the heart.

101. A: The ventricles are the chambers of the heart that pump blood; the right ventricle pumps deoxygenated blood to the lungs and the left oxygenated blood to the rest of the body. The atria are the chambers of the heart that receive blood. The endocardium covers the inner layer of the heart; the septum is the wall of cartilage that separates the four chambers.

102. C: The human body has an average of 8 to 10 pints, or 4 to 5 quarts, of blood.

103. D: Approximately 92% of plasma is composed of water; the remainder is composed of solutes. Fibrinogen is a plasma protein; electrolytes such as sodium, calcium, and potassium come from food and are found in plasma in smaller amounts.

104. C: Aspartate aminotransferase (AST) is typically used to diagnose cardiovascular conditions. Hemoglobin (Hgb), complete blood count (CBC), and erythrocyte sedimentation rate (ESR) are used to diagnose blood diseases such as anemia or leukemia.

105. B: The arterial puncture site is typically used for testing arterial blood gases (ABGs); the antecubital veins are used for venipuncture, with the median cubital vein considered the first choice. The veins located in the antecubital fossa are used for venous puncture.

106. C: A suprapubic specimen may be collected for infants or small children to ensure that the sample is not contaminated; the clean catch and midstream clean catch methods are used for adults to ensure an uncontaminated specimen. For a regular void specimen, urine is simply collected in a wide-mouth container.

107. D: Tests for cerebrospinal fluid (CSF) include total protein, glucose, and chloride; ABO typing is used for paternity testing.

108. B: A postprandial (PP) specimen is collected 2 hours after ingestion of a meal; fasting blood sugar (FBS) testing occurs after the patient has fasted 12 hours. Hgb, or hemoglobin, may be collected regardless of meals. HBV stands for hepatitis B virus.

109. A: Alcohol, corticosteroids, blood pressure medications, or birth control pills may affect the results of the glucose tolerance test (GTT); aspirin does not affect GTT results.

110. B: Activated coagulation time (ACT), prothrombin time (PT), and partial thromboplastin time (PTT) are all used for coagulation monitoring; Hgb, or hemoglobin, is used for the diagnosis of anemia.

111. C: The prothrombin time (PT) test may be used in conjunction with partial thromboplastin time (PTT) to assess a patient's total clotting abnormalities;

activated coagulation time (ACT) is used to monitor heparin therapy. APPT stands for activated partial thromboplastin time and PP postprandial testing.

112. B: As with prothrombin time (PT), activated partial thromboplastin time (APPT) whole blood values differ from plasma values; normal whole blood values range from 93 to 127 seconds and normal plasma values from 24 to 34 seconds.

113. A: Blood gas values such as partial pressure of carbon dioxide (pCO_2) are typically ordered stat; human chorionic gonadotropin (HCG) is a pregnancy test. The fasting blood sugar (FBS) test is a timed test for which patients must restrict dietary intake for 12 hours. The hemoglobin (Hgb) test is used to diagnose anemia.

114. C: Enteric isolation procedures are required for patients with intestinal infections that may be transmitted by ingestion; drainage/secretion isolation is required for burn patients or those with skin infections. AFB (acid-fast-bacilli) isolation is used for patients with tuberculosis.

115. D: The Occupational Safety and Health Administration (OSHA) requires that a high-efficiency particulate air (HEPA) respirator be used to protect healthcare workers caring for acid-fast-bacilli (AFB) patients, such as those with infectious tuberculosis; a HEPA respirator is not required for enteric or contact isolation patients or burn patients.

116. C: The Occupational Safety and Health Administration (OSHA) requires manufacturers of hazardous chemicals to supply safety data sheets (SDS) for all chemical products; SDS are kept in a laboratory logbook or binder as a reference for lab personnel.

117. A: Contaminated needles should never be recapped; the phlebotomist should replace the patient's bed rails after specimen collection and report unusual odors, spills, or dropped items to the nurse.

118. C: Environmental conditions such as water, oxygen or lack of oxygen, proper pH, darkness, and proper temperature of 37.5ºC or 98.6ºF are required for pathogen growth.

119. B: Postexposure treatment with hepatitis B immune globulin (HBIG) is effective in preventing HBV; however, no vaccine is available for either HCV or HIV.

120. C: Because exposure does not necessarily lead to human immunodeficiency virus (HIV), as well as the potential for serious drug side effects, postexposure treatment is not recommended for all occupational exposures to HIV. No vaccine is available for HIV, and HIV may be transmitted through breast milk. Those exposed to HIV should be tested 6 weeks, 12 weeks, and 6 months after exposure.

121. B: The reservoir host is a person, animal, plant, or other organism or substance that acts as the source of transmission of a pathogen; the susceptible host is the person capable of being infected with a pathogen. The chain of infection is the order in which pathogens are transmitted; direct contact is the direct physical transfer of pathogens from a reservoir to a susceptible host.

122. D: Personal protective equipment (PPE) such as gloves, mask, and gowns is required when entering the room of a patient under drainage/secretion isolation, such as those with skin infections, AFB isolation, such as those with tuberculosis, or enteric isolation, such as those with intestinal infections that may be transmitted through ingestion; PPE is not required for patients with HIV.

123. C: Some chemicals may be activated by water and should not be flushed; the safety data sheets (SDS) should be consulted for detailed information regarding antidotes. Mixing bleach and ammonia creates a gas that may be toxic. Electrical hazards should be moved away from the patient using a broom handle or another object made of glass or wood. Lead aprons and lead-lined gloves are required as a precaution against radioactive hazards.

124. B: The accession number, time of test, patient's name and date of birth, and the phlebotomist's initials are required information on specimen tube labels; the physician's signature is required on requisition forms.

125. D: Laboratory requisition forms may be transmitted to the laboratory via courier, pneumatic tube system, or in the case of computerized forms, e-mail; verbal laboratory requests may only be given in the outpatient or emergency setting and must be documented on a laboratory requisition form.

126. B: When taking calls, the phlebotomist should not wait until the first call is finished before taking another call; ask the first caller for permission to be put on hold, then answer the second call. When the second call is completed, return to the

first call. An individual's "personal space," or comfort zone, is based on culture and should be respected. Sign language may be used for both hearing-impaired and non–English-speaking patients.

127. C: Negligence is defined as the failure to act, resulting in injury or harm to the patient, and does not require intent to harm. Invasion of privacy is a tort involving use of a patient's name for commercial gain, intrusion into a patient's private life, or disclosure of private information. Abandonment is the premature termination of a professional relationship with a patient without notice or patient consent.

128. A: Abandonment, or the premature termination of a professional relationship between a healthcare provider and a patient without notice or patient consent, is an example of an intentional tort; negligence does not require intent. Malpractice is negligence or improper treatment by a health care professional. Chain of custody refers to the procedure for ensuring that specimens have been obtained for the correct patient, have been labeled correctly, and have not been subject to tampering.

129. C: Pre- and post- are examples of a prefix, which is added to the beginning of a word to indicate an amount, location, or time; pre- means "before" and post- means "after." A suffix is added to the end of a word and indicates a procedure, condition, or disease, such as "-algia," or pain. An abbreviation is used to shorten a medical term, such as "BID," or twice a day. A root word is the basis of a term and establishes its meaning; for example, "cardi" is a root word meaning heart.

130. D: The term caudal means toward the tail, or inferior; cranial means toward the head, or superior. The term medial means toward the midline, and lateral means toward the side of the body.

131. C: Glass tubes are preferred for blood alcohol specimens because of the porous nature of plastic tubes; random drug screening may be performed without patient consent, such as in the case of athletes or employees of health care organizations. A split sample may be required for confirmation or parallel testing. A proctor may be required to be present to verify that the specimen was obtained from the correct individual.

132. A: Failing to maintain blood pressure at 40 mm Hg may decrease bleeding time; aspirin, ethanol, dextran, or other drugs containing salicylate may prolong bleeding time.

133. B: The activated clotting time (ACT) test is used to monitor heparin levels; partial pressure of oxygen (PO_2) is an arterial blood gas and ionized calcium an electrolyte. Glucose levels are measured by the 2-hour postprandial (PP) test.

134. D: Arsenic, zinc, iron, copper, aluminum, and lead are all examples of trace elements; magnesium is not a trace element.

135. B: Measurement of cardiac troponin is useful in the diagnosis of acute myocardial infarction or heart attack; glucose testing is used in diagnosing diabetes. Hematocrit is used for anemia and occult blood for colon cancer screening.

136. C: B-type natriuretic peptide (BNP) blood concentrations are measured to detect congestive heart failure; the purified protein derivative (PPD) skin test is used to test for tuberculosis. The Histo and Cocci skin tests are used to test for the fungal infections *Histoplasmosis* and *Coccidioidomycosis*, respectively.

137. B: In administering a tuberculosis (TB) skin test, the antigen should be injected just below the skin, not into a vein. Presence of a bleb or wheal indicates that the antigen was injected properly. A TB reaction is measured according to the degree of induration or hardness, not erythema or redness.

138. C: A positive reaction to a TB skin test is indicated by induration of 10 mm or greater in diameter; induration between 5 and 9 mm in diameter indicates a doubtful reaction and less than 5 mm in diameter a negative reaction. The degree of redness or erythema is not relevant.

139. D: The first step in performing a test for group A streptococci is nitrous acid or enzymatic extraction of the throat swab specimen, followed by latex agglutination or enzyme immunoassay for antigen detection. Specific gravity is measured through urinalysis.

140. C: Arterial puncture is primarily performed to evaluate arterial blood gasses (ABGs). Arterial puncture is usually more difficult to perform and more painful than venipuncture; thus, it is not used for routine blood tests.

141. B: PO_2, or partial pressure of oxygen, is used to measure oxygen levels in the blood; decreased oxygen levels increase the respiration rate and vice versa. PCO_2, or

partial pressure of carbon dioxide, is used to measure carbon dioxide levels in the blood; increased CO_2 levels in the blood increase the respiration rate and vice versa. HCO_3 measures the amount of bicarbonate in the blood and is used to evaluate the bicarbonate system in the kidneys. pH measures the acidity or alkalinity of the blood.

142. D: Base excess or deficit is used to calculate the nonrespiratory part of acid-base balance and is based on PCO_2, HCO_3, and hematocrit (Hct) levels; O_2 saturation is the percentage of oxygen bound to hemoglobin.

143. D: Because the radial artery can be easily compressed over the wrist, it carries a lower risk of hematoma; however, because of its small size, it may be difficult to locate in patients with low cardiac output. If the radial artery is damaged during arterial puncture, the ulnar artery may be used to supply blood to the hand. The radial artery should not be punctured in the absence of collateral circulation.

144. A: The femoral artery is located in the groin and is usually used for arterial puncture only in emergency situations or when no other sites are available; arterial specimens may also be obtained from the scalp or from the umbilical arteries in infants. The brachial artery is located in the arm near the insertion of the biceps muscle.

145. C: The Allen test is used to assess collateral circulation. In performing the Allen test, both the radial and ulnar arteries should be compressed at the same time to assess the return of blood when pressure is released. The patient should not hyperextend the fingers when opening his or her hand because this may result in decreased blood flow and interfere with results. A positive result is indicated when the hand flushes pink or returns to normal color within 15 seconds.

146. B: In infants, the scalp or umbilical artery may be used for arterial puncture. The brachial artery is not used in infants or children because it is more difficult to palpate and lacks collateral circulation. The femoral artery is generally only used in emergency situations or if no other sites are available. The ulnar artery is not used for arterial puncture.

147. A: The presence of a bleb or wheal indicates proper injection of a local anesthetic prior to arterial puncture as well as proper injection of the antigen during tuberculosis (TB) testing. Induration or hardness of 10 mm or greater

indicates a positive TB reaction. A positive Allen test is indicated by the hand flushing pink or regaining normal coloration within 15 seconds.

148. C: The vasovagal response is fainting or loss of consciousness due to a nervous system response to abrupt pain or trauma, and may occur during arterial puncture. A hematoma is the appearance of swelling or a blood mass during or following venipuncture. Myocardial infarction is also known as heart attack.

149. D: Serous fluid may be obtained from the peritoneal or abdominal cavity, the pleural cavity surrounding the lungs, or the pericardial cavity surrounding the heart. Cerebrospinal fluid is obtained from the spinal cavity.

150. B: The C-urea breath test is used to detect the presence of *Helicobacter pylori*, a form of bacteria causing chronic gastritis and eventually leading to peptic ulcer; the hydrogen breath test is used to assess lactose intolerance. Bone marrow biopsy is used to test for blood disorders and hair samples to detect trace or heavy metals.

Special Report: High Frequency Terms

The following terms were compiled as high frequency Phlebotomy test terms. I recommend printing out this list and identifying the terms you are unfamiliar with. Then, use a medical dictionary or the internet to look up the terms you have questions about. Take one section per day if you have the time to maximize recall.

A

Acquired immunodeficiency syndrome
Amenorrhea
Aneurysm
Angina pectoris
Angiogenesis
Anklyosing spondylitis
Anxiety
Appendicitis
Arterial disease
Arteriosclerosis
Arthralgia
Arthritis
Atypical angina
AZT

B

Back pain
Blood cultures
Bradycardia
Braxton-Hicks contractions
Bronchiectasis
Bulimia

C

CAD
Cancer
Candidiasis
Cardiac disease

Carpal tunnel syndrome
Chest pain
Chest x-ray
Cirrhosis
COLD
Corticosteroids

D

Degenerative heart disease
Diabetes insipidus
Diabetes mellitus
Diabetic nephropathy
Dialysis
Diaphoresis
Down's syndrome
DVT
Dyspnea

E

Ectopic pregnancy
Electrocardiogram (ECG)
Embolism
Emphysema
Endocrine system
Epinephrine
Esophagitis

F

Fallopian tube
Fatigue
Fecal incontinence
Fibrillation
Fibromyalgia syndrome

G

Gangrene
Glucagon
Glucose tolerance test
Guillai-Barre' syndrome

H

Heart failure
Heart rate
Hemophilia
Hemorrhage
Heparin
Hepatitis (A-E)
Herpes zoster
Hiatal hernia
HIV
Hyponatremia
Hypothyroidism
Hypoxia
Hysterectomy

I

Immune serum globulin
Induration
Inflammatory bowel disease
Inhibitors
Interferon
Ischemic Heart Disease

J

Jaundice
Joint pain
Joint sepsis
Jevenile rheumatoid arthritis

K

Kidney failure
Kidney stones

L

Labile hypertension
Lactation
Low back pain
Lymphocyctes

M

Macrophages
Menarche
Ménière's disease
Metabolism
Multiple sclerosis
Myalgias

N

Neck pain
Neomycin
Night sweats
Nitrates
Nitroglycerin
Nocturnal angina
Norepinephrine
Nystagmus

O

Orthostatic hypotension
Osteoarthritis
Osteoporosis

P

Pain–joint
Palmar erythema
Palpitations
Pancreatitis
Parathyroid hormone
Paresthesia
Parkinson's disease
Pelvic inflammatory disease (PID)
Pericarditis
Pregnancy
Psychological support
Pulmonary edema

Q

Quadriceps

R

RA- Rheumatoid arthritis
Referred pain
Renal failure
Respiration
Rheumatic fever
Right ventricular failure

S

Sciatica
Scleroderma
Serotonin
Serum cholesterol
Sex hormones
Shoulder pain
Sickle cell anemia
Sinus bradycardia

Sinus tachycardia
Smoking
Systolic rate

T

Tendinitis
Thyroid gland
Tissue necrosis
Trauma
Tuberculosis

U

Ulceration
Umbilical pain
Ureter obstruction
Urethritis
Urinary bladder
Urinary tract infection

V

Vaginal bleeding
Vaginal lubricant
Ventricular failure
Vertigo
Vital signs
Vomiting

W

Weight gain

Special Report: Difficult Patients

Every phlebotomist will eventually get a difficult patient on their list of responsibilities. These patients can be mentally, physically, and emotionally combative in many different environments. Consequently, care of these patients should be conducted in a manner for personal and self-protection of the phlebotomist. Some of the key guidelines are as follows:

1. Never allow yourself to be cornered in a room with the patient positioned between you and the door.
2. Don't escalate the tension with verbal bantering. Basically, don't argue with the patient or resident.
3. Ask permission before performing any normal tasks in a patient's room whenever possible.
4. Discuss your concerns with the nursing staff. Consult the floor supervisor if necessary, especially when safety is an issue.
5. Get help from other support staff when offering care. Get a witness if you are anticipating abuse of any kind.
6. Remove yourself from the situation if you are concerned about your personal safety at all times.
7. If attacked, defend yourself with the force necessary for self-protection and attempt to separate from the patient.
8. Be aware of the patient's medical and mental history prior to entering the patient's room.
9. Don't put yourself in a position to be hurt.
10. Get the necessary help for all transfers, bathing and dressing activities from other staff members for difficult patients.
11. Respect the resident and patient's personal property.
12. Get assistance quickly, via the call bell or vocal projection, if a situation becomes violent or abuse.
13. Immediately seek medical treatment if injured.
14. Fill out an incident report for proper documentation of the occurrence.
15. Protect other patients from abusive behavior.

Special Report: Guidelines for Standard Precautions

Standard precautions are precautions taken to avoid contracting various diseases and preventing the spread of disease to those who have compromised immunity. Some of these diseases include human immunodeficiency virus (HIV), acquired immunodeficiency syndrome (AIDS), and hepatitis B (HBV). Standard precautions are needed since many diseases do not display signs or symptoms in their early stages. Standard precautions mean to treat all body fluids/ substances as if they were contaminated. These body fluids include but are not limited to the following blood, semen, vaginal secretions, breast milk, amniotic fluid, feces, urine, peritoneal fluid, synovial fluid, cerebrospinal fluid, secretions from the nasal and oral cavities, and lacrimal and sweat gland excretions. This means that standard precautions should be used with all patients.

1. A shield for the eyes and face must be used if there is a possibility of splashes from blood and body fluids.
2. If possibility of blood or body fluids being splashed on clothing, you must wear a plastic apron.
3. Gloves must be worn if you could possibly come in contact with blood or body fluids. They are also needed if you are going to touch something that may have come in contact with blood or body fluids.
4. Hands must be washed even if you were wearing gloves. Hands must be washed and gloves must be changed between patients. Wash hands with at a dime size amount of soap and warm water for about 30 seconds. Singing "Mary had a little lamb" is approximately 30 seconds.
5. Blood and body fluid spills must be cleansed and disinfected using a solution of one part bleach to 10 parts water or your hospital's accepted method.
6. Used needles must be separated from clean needles. Throw both the needle and the syringe away in the sharps' container. The sharps' container is made of puncture proof material.
7. Take extra care in performing high-risk activities that include puncturing the skin and cutting the skin.
8. CPR equipment to be used in a hospital must include resuscitation bags and mouthpieces.

Special precautions must be taken to dispose of biomedical waste. Biomedical waste includes but is not limited to the following: laboratory waste, pathology waste, liquid waste from suction, all sharp object, bladder catheters, chest tubes, IV tubes, and drainage containers. Biomedical waste is removed from a facility by trained biomedical waste disposers.

The health care professional is legally and ethically responsible for adhering to standard precautions. They may prevent you from contracting a fatal disease or from a patient contracting a disease from you that could be deadly.

CPR Review/Cheat Sheet

Topic	New Guidelines
Conscious Choking	5 back blows, then 5 abdominal thrusts- adult/child
Unconscious Choking	5 chest compressions, look, 2 breaths-adult/child/infant
Rescue Breaths	Normal Breath given over 1 second until chest rises
Chest Compressions to Ventilation Ratios (Single Rescuer)	30:2 – Adult/Child/Infant
Chest Compressions to Ventilation Ratios (Two Rescuer)	30:2 – Adult 15:2 – Child/Infant
Chest Compression rate	About 100/minute – Adult/Child/Infant
Chest Compression Land marking Method	Simplified approach – center of the chest – Adult/Child 2 or 3 fingers, just below the nipple line at the center of the chest - Infant
AED	1 shock, then 2 minutes (or 5 cycles) of CPR
Anaphylaxis	Assist person with use of prescribed auto injector
Asthma	Assist person with use of prescribed inhaler

- Check the scene
- Check for responsiveness – ask, "Are you OK?"
- Adult - call 911, then administer CPR
- Child/Infant – administer CPR for 5 cycles, then call 911
- Open victim's airway and check for breathing – look, listen, and feel for 5 - 10 seconds
- Two rescue breaths should be given, 1 second each, and should produce a visible chest rise
- If the air does not go in, reposition and try 2 breaths again
- Check victim's pulse – chest compressions are recommended if an infant or child has a rate less than 60 per minute with signs of poor perfusion.
- Begin 30 compressions to 2 breaths at a rate of 1 breath every 5 seconds for Adult; 1 breath every 3 seconds for child/infant
- Continue 30:2 ratio until victim moves, AED is brought to the scene, or professional help arrives

AED

- ADULT/ Child over 8 years old - use Adult pads
- Child 1-8 years old – use Child pads or use Adult pads by placing one on the chest and one on the back of the child
- Infant under 1 year of age - AED not recommended

Secret Key #1 - Time is Your Greatest Enemy

Pace Yourself

Wear a watch. At the beginning of the test, check the time (or start a chronometer on your watch to count the minutes), and check the time after every few questions to make sure you are "on schedule."

If you are forced to speed up, do it efficiently. Usually one or more answer choices can be eliminated without too much difficulty. Above all, don't panic. Don't speed up and just begin guessing at random choices. By pacing yourself, and continually monitoring your progress against your watch, you will always know exactly how far ahead or behind you are with your available time. If you find that you are one minute behind on the test, don't skip one question without spending any time on it, just to catch back up. Take 15 fewer seconds on the next four questions, and after four questions you'll have caught back up. Once you catch back up, you can continue working each problem at your normal pace.

Furthermore, don't dwell on the problems that you were rushed on. If a problem was taking up too much time and you made a hurried guess, it must be difficult. The difficult questions are the ones you are most likely to miss anyway, so it isn't a big loss. It is better to end with more time than you need than to run out of time.

Lastly, sometimes it is beneficial to slow down if you are constantly getting ahead of time. You are always more likely to catch a careless mistake by working more slowly than quickly, and among very high-scoring test takers (those who are likely to have lots of time left over), careless errors affect the score more than mastery of material.

Secret Key #2 - Guessing is not Guesswork

You probably know that guessing is a good idea. Unlike other standardized tests, there is no penalty for getting a wrong answer. Even if you have no idea about a question, you still have a 20-25% chance of getting it right.

Most test takers do not understand the impact that proper guessing can have on their score. Unless you score extremely high, guessing will significantly contribute to your final score.

Monkeys Take the Test

What most test takers don't realize is that to insure that 20-25% chance, you have to guess randomly. If you put 20 monkeys in a room to take this test, assuming they answered once per question and behaved themselves, on average they would get 20-25% of the questions correct. Put 20 test takers in the room, and the average will be much lower among guessed questions. Why?
1. The test writers intentionally write deceptive answer choices that "look" right. A test taker has no idea about a question, so he picks the "best looking" answer, which is often wrong. The monkey has no idea what looks good and what doesn't, so it will consistently be right about 20-25% of the time.
2. Test takers will eliminate answer choices from the guessing pool based on a hunch or intuition. Simple but correct answers often get excluded, leaving a 0% chance of being correct. The monkey has no clue, and often gets lucky with the best choice.

This is why the process of elimination endorsed by most test courses is flawed and detrimental to your performance. Test takers don't guess; they make an ignorant stab in the dark that is usually worse than random.

$5 Challenge

Let me introduce one of the most valuable ideas of this course—the $5 challenge:

You only mark your "best guess" if you are willing to bet $5 on it.
You only eliminate choices from guessing if you are willing to bet $5 on it.

Why $5? Five dollars is an amount of money that is small yet not insignificant, and can really add up fast (20 questions could cost you $100). Likewise, each answer choice on one question of the test will have a small impact on your overall score, but it can really add up to a lot of points in the end.

The process of elimination IS valuable. The following shows your chance of guessing it right:

If you eliminate wrong answer choices until only this many remain:	Chance of getting it correct:
1	100%
2	50%
3	33%

However, if you accidentally eliminate the right answer or go on a hunch for an incorrect answer, your chances drop dramatically—to 0%. By guessing among all the answer choices, you are GUARANTEED to have a shot at the right answer.

That's why the $5 test is so valuable. If you give up the advantage and safety of a pure guess, it had better be worth the risk.

What we still haven't covered is how to be sure that whatever guess you make is truly random. Here's the easiest way:

Always pick the first answer choice among those remaining.

Such a technique means that you have decided, **before you see a single test question**, exactly how you are going to guess, and since the order of choices tells you nothing about which one is correct, this guessing technique is perfectly random.

This section is not meant to scare you away from making educated guesses or eliminating choices; you just need to define when a choice is worth eliminating. The $5 test, along with a pre-defined random guessing strategy, is the best way to make sure you reap all of the benefits of guessing.

Secret Key #3 - Practice Smarter, Not Harder

Many test takers delay the test preparation process because they dread the awful amounts of practice time they think necessary to succeed on the test. We have refined an effective method that will take you only a fraction of the time.

There are a number of "obstacles" in the path to success. Among these are answering questions, finishing in time, and mastering test-taking strategies. All must be executed on the day of the test at peak performance, or your score will suffer. The test is a mental marathon that has a large impact on your future.

Just like a marathon runner, it is important to work your way up to the full challenge. So first you just worry about questions, and then time, and finally strategy:

Success Strategy

1. Find a good source for practice tests.
2. If you are willing to make a larger time investment, consider using more than one study guide. Often the different approaches of multiple authors will help you "get" difficult concepts.
3. Take a practice test with no time constraints, with all study helps, "open book." Take your time with questions and focus on applying strategies.
4. Take a practice test with time constraints, with all guides, "open book."
5. Take a final practice test without open material and with time limits.

If you have time to take more practice tests, just repeat step 5. By gradually exposing yourself to the full rigors of the test environment, you will condition your mind to the stress of test day and maximize your success.

Secret Key #4 - Prepare, Don't Procrastinate

Let me state an obvious fact: if you take the test three times, you will probably get three different scores. This is due to the way you feel on test day, the level of preparedness you have, and the version of the test you see. Despite the test writers' claims to the contrary, some versions of the test WILL be easier for you than others.

Since your future depends so much on your score, you should maximize your chances of success. In order to maximize the likelihood of success, you've got to prepare in advance. This means taking practice tests and spending time learning the information and test taking strategies you will need to succeed.

Never go take the actual test as a "practice" test, expecting that you can just take it again if you need to. Take all the practice tests you can on your own, but when you go to take the official test, be prepared, be focused, and do your best the first time!

Secret Key #5 - Test Yourself

Everyone knows that time is money. There is no need to spend too much of your time or too little of your time preparing for the test. You should only spend as much of your precious time preparing as is necessary for you to get the score you need.

Once you have taken a practice test under real conditions of time constraints, then you will know if you are ready for the test or not.

If you have scored extremely high the first time that you take the practice test, then there is not much point in spending countless hours studying. You are already there.

Benchmark your abilities by retaking practice tests and seeing how much you have improved. Once you consistently score high enough to guarantee success, then you are ready.

If you have scored well below where you need, then knuckle down and begin studying in earnest. Check your improvement regularly through the use of practice tests under real conditions. Above all, don't worry, panic, or give up. The key is perseverance!

Then, when you go to take the test, remain confident and remember how well you did on the practice tests. If you can score high enough on a practice test, then you can do the same on the real thing.

General Strategies

The most important thing you can do is to ignore your fears and jump into the test immediately. Do not be overwhelmed by any strange-sounding terms. You have to jump into the test like jumping into a pool—all at once is the easiest way.

Make Predictions

As you read and understand the question, try to guess what the answer will be. Remember that several of the answer choices are wrong, and once you begin reading them, your mind will immediately become cluttered with answer choices designed to throw you off. Your mind is typically the most focused immediately after you have read the question and digested its contents. If you can, try to predict what the correct answer will be. You may be surprised at what you can predict.

Quickly scan the choices and see if your prediction is in the listed answer choices. If it is, then you can be quite confident that you have the right answer. It still won't hurt to check the other answer choices, but most of the time, you've got it!

Answer the Question

It may seem obvious to only pick answer choices that answer the question, but the test writers can create some excellent answer choices that are wrong. Don't pick an answer just because it sounds right, or you believe it to be true. It MUST answer the question. Once you've made your selection, always go back and check it against the question and make sure that you didn't misread the question and that the answer choice does answer the question posed.

Benchmark

After you read the first answer choice, decide if you think it sounds correct or not. If it doesn't, move on to the next answer choice. If it does, mentally mark that answer choice. This doesn't mean that you've definitely selected it as your answer choice, it just means that it's the best you've seen thus far. Go ahead and read the next choice. If the next choice is worse than the one you've already selected, keep going to the next answer choice. If the next choice is better than the choice you've already selected, mentally mark the new answer choice as your best guess.

The first answer choice that you select becomes your standard. Every other answer choice must be benchmarked against that standard. That choice is correct until proven otherwise by another answer choice beating it out. Once you've decided that no other answer choice seems as good, do one final check to ensure that your answer choice answers the question posed.

Valid Information

Don't discount any of the information provided in the question. Every piece of information may be necessary to determine the correct answer. None of the information in the question is there to throw you off (while the answer choices will certainly have information to throw you off). If two seemingly unrelated topics are discussed, don't ignore either. You can be confident there is a relationship, or it wouldn't be included in the question, and you are probably going to have to determine what is that relationship to find the answer.

Avoid "Fact Traps"

Don't get distracted by a choice that is factually true. Your search is for the answer that answers the question. Stay focused and don't fall for an answer that is true but irrelevant. Always go back to the question and make sure you're choosing an answer that actually answers the question and is not just a true statement. An answer can be factually correct, but it MUST answer the question asked. Additionally, two answers can both be seemingly correct, so be sure to read all of the answer choices, and make sure that you get the one that BEST answers the question.

Milk the Question

Some of the questions may throw you completely off. They might deal with a subject you have not been exposed to, or one that you haven't reviewed in years. While your lack of knowledge about the subject will be a hindrance, the question itself can give you many clues that will help you find the correct answer. Read the question carefully and look for clues. Watch particularly for adjectives and nouns describing difficult terms or words that you don't recognize. Regardless of whether you completely understand a word or not, replacing it with a synonym, either provided or one you more familiar with, may help you to understand what the questions are asking. Rather than wracking your mind about specific detailed information concerning a difficult term or word, try to use mental substitutes that are easier to understand.

The Trap of Familiarity

Don't just choose a word because you recognize it. On difficult questions, you may not recognize a number of words in the answer choices. The test writers don't put "make-believe" words on the test, so don't think that just because you only recognize all the words in one answer choice that that answer choice must be correct. If you only recognize words in one answer choice, then focus on that one. Is it correct? Try your best to determine if it is correct. If it is, that's great. If not, eliminate it. Each word and answer choice you eliminate increases your chances of getting the question correct, even if you then have to guess among the unfamiliar choices.

Eliminate Answers

Eliminate choices as soon as you realize they are wrong. But be careful! Make sure you consider all of the possible answer choices. Just because one appears right, doesn't mean that the next one won't be even better! The test writers will usually put more than one good answer choice for every question, so read all of them. Don't worry if you are stuck between two that seem right. By getting down to just two remaining possible choices, your odds are now 50/50. Rather than wasting too much time, play the odds. You are guessing, but guessing wisely because you've been able to knock out some of the answer choices that you know are wrong. If you are eliminating choices and realize that the last answer choice you are left with is also obviously wrong, don't panic. Start over and consider each choice again. There may easily be something that you missed the first time and will realize on the second pass.

Tough Questions

If you are stumped on a problem or it appears too hard or too difficult, don't waste time. Move on! Remember though, if you can quickly check for obviously incorrect answer choices, your chances of guessing correctly are greatly improved. Before you completely give up, at least try to knock out a couple of possible answers. Eliminate what you can and then guess at the remaining answer choices before moving on.

Brainstorm

If you get stuck on a difficult question, spend a few seconds quickly brainstorming. Run through the complete list of possible answer choices. Look at each choice and ask yourself, "Could this answer the question satisfactorily?" Go through each answer choice and consider it independently of the others. By systematically going through all possibilities, you may find something that you would otherwise overlook. Remember though that when you get stuck, it's important to try to keep moving.

Read Carefully

Understand the problem. Read the question and answer choices carefully. Don't miss the question because you misread the terms. You have plenty of time to read each question thoroughly and make sure you understand what is being asked. Yet a happy medium must be attained, so don't waste too much time. You must read carefully, but efficiently.

Face Value

When in doubt, use common sense. Always accept the situation in the problem at face value. Don't read too much into it. These problems will not require you to make huge leaps of logic. The test writers aren't trying to throw you off with a cheap trick. If you have to go beyond creativity and make a leap of logic in order to have an answer choice answer the question, then you should look at the other answer choices. Don't overcomplicate the problem by creating theoretical relationships or explanations that will warp time or space. These are normal problems rooted in reality. It's just that the applicable relationship or explanation may not be readily apparent and you have to figure things out. Use your common sense to interpret anything that isn't clear.

Prefixes

If you're having trouble with a word in the question or answer choices, try dissecting it. Take advantage of every clue that the word might include. Prefixes and suffixes can be a huge help. Usually they allow you to determine a basic meaning. Pre- means before, post- means after, pro - is positive, de- is negative. From these prefixes and suffixes, you can get an idea of the general meaning of the word and try to put it into context. Beware though of any traps. Just because con- is the opposite of pro-, doesn't necessarily mean congress is the opposite of progress!

Hedge Phrases

Watch out for critical hedge phrases, led off with words such as "likely," "may," "can," "sometimes," "often," "almost," "mostly," "usually," "generally," "rarely," and "sometimes." Question writers insert these hedge phrases to cover every possibility. Often an answer choice will be wrong simply because it leaves no room for exception. Unless the situation calls for them, avoid answer choices that have definitive words like "exactly," and "always."

Switchback Words

Stay alert for "switchbacks." These are the words and phrases frequently used to alert you to shifts in thought. The most common switchback word is "but." Others

- 128 -

include "although," "however," "nevertheless," "on the other hand," "even though," "while," "in spite of," "despite," and "regardless of."

New Information

Correct answer choices will rarely have completely new information included. Answer choices typically are straightforward reflections of the material asked about and will directly relate to the question. If a new piece of information is included in an answer choice that doesn't even seem to relate to the topic being asked about, then that answer choice is likely incorrect. All of the information needed to answer the question is usually provided for you in the question. You should not have to make guesses that are unsupported or choose answer choices that require unknown information that cannot be reasoned from what is given.

Time Management

On technical questions, don't get lost on the technical terms. Don't spend too much time on any one question. If you don't know what a term means, then odds are you aren't going to get much further since you don't have a dictionary. You should be able to immediately recognize whether or not you know a term. If you don't, work with the other clues that you have—the other answer choices and terms provided—but don't waste too much time trying to figure out a difficult term that you don't know.

Contextual Clues

Look for contextual clues. An answer can be right but not the correct answer. The contextual clues will help you find the answer that is most right and is correct. Understand the context in which a phrase or statement is made. This will help you make important distinctions.

Don't Panic

Panicking will not answer any questions for you; therefore, it isn't helpful. When you first see the question, if your mind goes blank, take a deep breath. Force yourself to mechanically go through the steps of solving the problem using the strategies you've learned.

Pace Yourself

Don't get clock fever. It's easy to be overwhelmed when you're looking at a page full of questions, your mind is full of random thoughts and feeling confused, and the clock is ticking down faster than you would like. Calm down and maintain the pace that you have set for yourself. As long as you are on track by monitoring your pace, you are guaranteed to have enough time for yourself. When you get to the last few minutes of the test, it may seem like you won't have enough time left, but if you only have as many questions as you should have left at that point, then you're right on track!

Answer Selection

The best way to pick an answer choice is to eliminate all of those that are wrong, until only one is left and confirm that is the correct answer. Sometimes though, an answer choice may immediately look right. Be careful! Take a second to make sure that the other choices are not equally obvious. Don't make a hasty mistake. There are only two times that you should stop before checking other answers. First is when you are positive that the answer choice you have selected is correct. Second is when time is almost out and you have to make a quick guess!

Check Your Work

Since you will probably not know every term listed and the answer to every question, it is important that you get credit for the ones that you do know. Don't miss any questions through careless mistakes. If at all possible, try to take a second to look back over your answer selection and make sure you've selected the correct answer choice and haven't made a costly careless mistake (such as marking an answer choice that you didn't mean to mark). The time it takes for this quick double check should more than pay for itself in caught mistakes.

Beware of Directly Quoted Answers

Sometimes an answer choice will repeat word for word a portion of the question or reference section. However, beware of such exact duplication. It may be a trap! More than likely, the correct choice will paraphrase or summarize a point, rather than being exactly the same wording.

Slang

Scientific sounding answers are better than slang ones. An answer choice that begins "To compare the outcomes…" is much more likely to be correct than one that begins "Because some people insisted…"

Extreme Statements

Avoid wild answers that throw out highly controversial ideas that are proclaimed as established fact. An answer choice that states the "process should used in certain situations, if…" is much more likely to be correct than one that states the "process should be discontinued completely." The first is a calm rational statement and doesn't even make a definitive, uncompromising stance, using a hedge word "if" to provide wiggle room, whereas the second choice is a radical idea and far more extreme.

Answer Choice Families

When you have two or more answer choices that are direct opposites or parallels, one of them is usually the correct answer. For instance, if one answer choice states "x increases" and another answer choice states "x decreases" or "y increases," then those two or three answer choices are very similar in construction and fall into the same family of answer choices. A family of answer choices consists of two or three answer choices, very similar in construction, but often with directly opposite meanings. Usually the correct answer choice will be in that family of answer choices. The "odd man out" or answer choice that doesn't seem to fit the parallel construction of the other answer choices is more likely to be incorrect.

Special Report: How to Overcome Test Anxiety

The very nature of tests caters to some level of anxiety, nervousness, or tension, just as we feel for any important event that occurs in our lives. A little bit of anxiety or nervousness can be a good thing. It helps us with motivation, and makes achievement just that much sweeter. However, too much anxiety can be a problem, especially if it hinders our ability to function and perform.

"Test anxiety," is the term that refers to the emotional reactions that some test-takers experience when faced with a test or exam. Having a fear of testing and exams is based upon a rational fear, since the test-taker's performance can shape the course of an academic career. Nevertheless, experiencing excessive fear of examinations will only interfere with the test-taker's ability to perform and chance to be successful.

There are a large variety of causes that can contribute to the development and sensation of test anxiety. These include, but are not limited to, lack of preparation and worrying about issues surrounding the test.

Lack of Preparation

Lack of preparation can be identified by the following behaviors or situations:

Not scheduling enough time to study, and therefore cramming the night before the test or exam
Managing time poorly, to create the sensation that there is not enough time to do everything
Failing to organize the text information in advance, so that the study material consists of the entire text and not simply the pertinent information
Poor overall studying habits

Worrying, on the other hand, can be related to both the test taker, or many other factors around him/her that will be affected by the results of the test. These include worrying about:

Previous performances on similar exams, or exams in general

How friends and other students are achieving

The negative consequences that will result from a poor grade or failure

There are three primary elements to test anxiety. Physical components, which involve the same typical bodily reactions as those to acute anxiety (to be discussed below). Emotional factors have to do with fear or panic. Mental or cognitive issues concerning attention spans and memory abilities.

Physical Signals

There are many different symptoms of test anxiety, and these are not limited to mental and emotional strain. Frequently there are a range of physical signals that will let a test taker know that he/she is suffering from test anxiety. These bodily changes can include the following:

Perspiring

Sweaty palms

Wet, trembling hands

Nausea

Dry mouth

A knot in the stomach

Headache

Faintness

Muscle tension

Aching shoulders, back and neck

Rapid heart beat

Feeling too hot/cold

To recognize the sensation of test anxiety, a test-taker should monitor him/herself for the following sensations:

The physical distress symptoms as listed above

Emotional sensitivity, expressing emotional feelings such as the need to cry or laugh too much, or a sensation of anger or helplessness

A decreased ability to think, causing the test-taker to blank out or have racing thoughts that are hard to organize or control.

Though most students will feel some level of anxiety when faced with a test or exam, the majority can cope with that anxiety and maintain it at a manageable level. However, those who cannot are faced with a very real and very serious condition, which can and should be controlled for the immeasurable benefit of this sufferer.

Naturally, these sensations lead to negative results for the testing experience. The most common effects of test anxiety have to do with nervousness and mental blocking.

Nervousness

Nervousness can appear in several different levels:

The test-taker's difficulty, or even inability to read and understand the questions on the test
The difficulty or inability to organize thoughts to a coherent form
The difficulty or inability to recall key words and concepts relating to the testing questions (especially essays)
The receipt of poor grades on a test, though the test material was well known by the test taker

Conversely, a person may also experience mental blocking, which involves:

Blanking out on test questions
Only remembering the correct answers to the questions when the test has already finished.

Fortunately for test anxiety sufferers, beating these feelings, to a large degree, has to do with proper preparation. When a test taker has a feeling of preparedness, then anxiety will be dramatically lessened.

The first step to resolving anxiety issues is to distinguish which of the two types of anxiety are being suffered. If the anxiety is a direct result of a lack of preparation, this should be considered a normal reaction, and the anxiety level (as opposed to the test results) shouldn't be anything to worry about. However, if, when adequately prepared, the test-taker still panics, blanks out, or seems to overreact, this is not a fully rational reaction. While this can be considered normal too, there are many ways to combat and overcome these effects.

Remember that anxiety cannot be entirely eliminated, however, there are ways to minimize it, to make the anxiety easier to manage. Preparation is one of the best ways to minimize test anxiety. Therefore the following techniques are wise in order to best fight off any anxiety that may want to build.

To begin with, try to avoid cramming before a test, whenever it is possible. By trying to memorize an entire term's worth of information in one day, you'll be shocking your system, and not giving yourself a very good chance to absorb the information. This is an easy path to anxiety, so for those who suffer from test anxiety, cramming should not even be considered an option.

Instead of cramming, work throughout the semester to combine all of the material which is presented throughout the semester, and work on it gradually as the course goes by, making sure to master the main concepts first, leaving minor details for a week or so before the test.

To study for the upcoming exam, be sure to pose questions that may be on the examination, to gauge the ability to answer them by integrating the ideas from your texts, notes and lectures, as well as any supplementary readings.

If it is truly impossible to cover all of the information that was covered in that particular term, concentrate on the most important portions, that can be covered very well. Learn these concepts as best as possible, so that when the test comes, a goal can be made to use these concepts as presentations of your knowledge.

In addition to study habits, changes in attitude are critical to beating a struggle with test anxiety. In fact, an improvement of the perspective over the entire test-taking experience can actually help a test taker to enjoy studying and therefore improve the overall experience. Be certain not to overemphasize the significance of the grade - know that the result of the test is neither a reflection of self worth, nor is it a measure of intelligence; one grade will not predict a person's future success.

To improve an overall testing outlook, the following steps should be tried:

Keeping in mind that the most reasonable expectation for taking a test is to expect to try to demonstrate as much of what you know as you possibly can. Reminding ourselves that a test is only one test; this is not the only one, and there will be others.

The thought of thinking of oneself in an irrational, all-or-nothing term should be avoided at all costs.

A reward should be designated for after the test, so there's something to look forward to. Whether it be going to a movie, going out to eat, or simply visiting friends, schedule it in advance, and do it no matter what result is expected on the exam.

Test-takers should also keep in mind that the basics are some of the most important things, even beyond anti-anxiety techniques and studying. Never neglect the basic social, emotional and biological needs, in order to try to absorb information. In order to best achieve, these three factors must be held as just as important as the studying itself.

Study Steps

Remember the following important steps for studying:

Maintain healthy nutrition and exercise habits. Continue both your recreational activities and social pass times. These both contribute to your physical and emotional well being.

Be certain to get a good amount of sleep, especially the night before the test, because when you're overtired you are not able to perform to the best of your best ability.

Keep the studying pace to a moderate level by taking breaks when they are needed, and varying the work whenever possible, to keep the mind fresh instead of getting bored.

When enough studying has been done that all the material that can be learned has been learned, and the test taker is prepared for the test, stop studying and do something relaxing such as listening to music, watching a movie, or taking a warm bubble bath.

There are also many other techniques to minimize the uneasiness or apprehension that is experienced along with test anxiety before, during, or even after the examination. In fact, there are a great deal of things that can be done to stop anxiety from interfering with lifestyle and performance. Again, remember that anxiety will not be eliminated entirely, and it shouldn't be. Otherwise that "up" feeling for exams would not exist, and most of us depend on that sensation to perform better than usual. However, this anxiety has to be at a level that is manageable.

Of course, as we have just discussed, being prepared for the exam is half the battle right away. Attending all classes, finding out what knowledge will be expected on the exam, and knowing the exam schedules are easy steps to lowering anxiety. Keeping up with work will remove the need to cram, and efficient study habits will eliminate wasted time. Studying should be done in an ideal location for concentration, so that it is simple to become interested in the material and give it complete attention. A method such as SQ3R (Survey, Question, Read, Recite, Review) is a wonderful key to follow to make sure that the study habits are as effective as possible, especially in the case of learning from a textbook. Flashcards are great techniques for memorization. Learning to take good notes will mean that notes will be full of useful information, so that less sifting will need to be done to seek out what is pertinent for studying. Reviewing notes after class and then again on occasion will keep the information fresh in the mind. From notes that have been taken summary sheets and outlines can be made for simpler reviewing.

A study group can also be a very motivational and helpful place to study, as there will be a sharing of ideas, all of the minds can work together, to make sure that everyone understands, and the studying will be made more interesting because it will be a social occasion.

Basically, though, as long as the test-taker remains organized and self confident, with efficient study habits, less time will need to be spent studying, and higher grades will be achieved.

To become self confident, there are many useful steps. The first of these is "self talk." It has been shown through extensive research, that self-talk for students who suffer from test anxiety, should be well monitored, in order to make sure that it contributes to self confidence as opposed to sinking the student. Frequently the self talk of test-anxious students is negative or self-defeating, thinking that everyone else is smarter and faster, that they always mess up, and that if they don't do well, they'll fail the entire course. It is important to decreasing anxiety that awareness is made of self talk. Try writing any negative self thoughts and then disputing them with a positive statement instead. Begin self-encouragement as though it was a friend speaking. Repeat positive statements to help reprogram the mind to believing in successes instead of failures.

Helpful Techniques

Other extremely helpful techniques include:

Self-visualization of doing well and reaching goals
While aiming for an "A" level of understanding, don't try to "overprotect" by setting your expectations lower. This will only convince the mind to stop studying in order to meet the lower expectations.
Don't make comparisons with the results or habits of other students. These are individual factors, and different things work for different people, causing different results.
Strive to become an expert in learning what works well, and what can be done in order to improve. Consider collecting this data in a journal.
Create rewards for after studying instead of doing things before studying that will only turn into avoidance behaviors.
Make a practice of relaxing - by using methods such as progressive relaxation, self-hypnosis, guided imagery, etc - in order to make relaxation an automatic sensation.
Work on creating a state of relaxed concentration so that concentrating will take on the focus of the mind, so that none will be wasted on worrying.
Take good care of the physical self by eating well and getting enough sleep.
Plan in time for exercise and stick to this plan.

Beyond these techniques, there are other methods to be used before, during and after the test that will help the test-taker perform well in addition to overcoming anxiety.

Before the exam comes the academic preparation. This involves establishing a study schedule and beginning at least one week before the actual date of the test. By doing this, the anxiety of not having enough time to study for the test will be automatically eliminated. Moreover, this will make the studying a much more effective experience, ensuring that the learning will be an easier process. This relieves much undue pressure on the test-taker.

Summary sheets, note cards, and flash cards with the main concepts and examples of these main concepts should be prepared in advance of the actual studying time. A topic should never be eliminated from this process. By omitting a topic because it isn't expected to be on the test is only setting up the test-taker for anxiety should it actually appear on the exam. Utilize the course syllabus for laying out the topics that should be studied. Carefully go over the notes that were made in class, paying special attention to any of the issues that the professor took special care to emphasize while lecturing in class. In the textbooks, use the chapter review, or if possible, the chapter tests, to begin your review.

It may even be possible to ask the instructor what information will be covered on the exam, or what the format of the exam will be (for example, multiple choice, essay, free form, true-false). Additionally, see if it is possible to find out how many questions will be on the test. If a review sheet or sample test has been offered by the professor, make good use of it, above anything else, for the preparation for the test. Another great resource for getting to know the examination is reviewing tests from previous semesters. Use these tests to review, and aim to achieve a 100% score on each of the possible topics. With a few exceptions, the goal that you set for yourself is the highest one that you will reach.

Take all of the questions that were assigned as homework, and rework them to any other possible course material. The more problems reworked, the more skill and confidence will form as a result. When forming the solution to a problem, write out each of the steps. Don't simply do head work. By doing as many steps on paper as possible, much clarification and therefore confidence will be formed. Do this with as many homework problems as possible, before checking the answers. By checking the answer after each problem, a reinforcement will exist, that will not be on the exam. Study situations should be as exam-like as possible, to prime the test-taker's system for the experience. By waiting to check the answers at the end, a psychological advantage will be formed, to decrease the stress factor.

Another fantastic reason for not cramming is the avoidance of confusion in concepts, especially when it comes to mathematics. 8-10 hours of study will become one hundred percent more effective if it is spread out over a week or at least several days, instead of doing it all in one sitting. Recognize that the human brain requires time in order to assimilate new material, so frequent breaks and a span of study time over several days will be much more beneficial.

Additionally, don't study right up until the point of the exam. Studying should stop a minimum of one hour before the exam begins. This allows the brain to rest and put things in their proper order. This will also provide the time to become as relaxed as possible when going into the examination room. The test-taker will also have time to eat well and eat sensibly. Know that the brain needs food as much as the rest of the body. With enough food and enough sleep, as well as a relaxed attitude, the body and the mind are primed for success.

Avoid any anxious classmates who are talking about the exam. These students only spread anxiety, and are not worth sharing the anxious sentimentalities.

Before the test also involves creating a positive attitude, so mental preparation should also be a point of concentration. There are many keys to creating a positive attitude. Should fears become rushing in, make a visualization of taking the exam, doing well, and seeing an A written on the paper. Write out a list of affirmations that will bring a feeling of confidence, such as "I am doing well in my English class," "I studied well and know my material," "I enjoy this class." Even if the affirmations aren't believed at first, it sends a positive message to the subconscious which will result in an alteration of the overall belief system, which is the system that creates reality.

If a sensation of panic begins, work with the fear and imagine the very worst! Work through the entire scenario of not passing the test, failing the entire course, and dropping out of school, followed by not getting a job, and pushing a shopping cart through the dark alley where you'll live. This will place things into perspective! Then, practice deep breathing and create a visualization of the opposite situation - achieving an "A" on the exam, passing the entire course, receiving the degree at a graduation ceremony.

On the day of the test, there are many things to be done to ensure the best results, as well as the most calm outlook. The following stages are suggested in order to maximize test-taking potential:

Begin the examination day with a moderate breakfast, and avoid any coffee or beverages with caffeine if the test taker is prone to jitters. Even people who are used to managing caffeine can feel jittery or light-headed when it is taken on a test day.

Attempt to do something that is relaxing before the examination begins. As last minute cramming clouds the mastering of overall concepts, it is better to use this time to create a calming outlook.

Be certain to arrive at the test location well in advance, in order to provide time to select a location that is away from doors, windows and other distractions, as well as giving enough time to relax before the test begins.

Keep away from anxiety generating classmates who will upset the sensation of stability and relaxation that is being attempted before the exam.

Should the waiting period before the exam begins cause anxiety, create a self-distraction by reading a light magazine or something else that is relaxing and simple.

During the exam itself, read the entire exam from beginning to end, and find out how much time should be allotted to each individual problem. Once writing the exam, should more time be taken for a problem, it should be abandoned, in order to begin another problem. If there is time at the end, the unfinished problem can always be returned to and completed.

Read the instructions very carefully - twice - so that unpleasant surprises won't follow during or after the exam has ended.

When writing the exam, pretend that the situation is actually simply the completion of homework within a library, or at home. This will assist in forming a relaxed atmosphere, and will allow the brain extra focus for the complex thinking function.

Begin the exam with all of the questions with which the most confidence is felt. This will build the confidence level regarding the entire exam and will begin a quality momentum. This will also create encouragement for trying the problems where uncertainty resides.

Going with the "gut instinct" is always the way to go when solving a problem. Second guessing should be avoided at all costs. Have confidence in the ability to do well.

For essay questions, create an outline in advance that will keep the mind organized and make certain that all of the points are remembered. For multiple choice, read every answer, even if the correct one has been spotted - a better one may exist.

Continue at a pace that is reasonable and not rushed, in order to be able to work carefully. Provide enough time to go over the answers at the end, to check for small errors that can be corrected.

Should a feeling of panic begin, breathe deeply, and think of the feeling of the body releasing sand through its pores. Visualize a calm, peaceful place, and include all of the sights, sounds and sensations of this image. Continue the deep breathing, and take a few minutes to continue this with closed eyes. When all is well again, return to the test.

If a "blanking" occurs for a certain question, skip it and move on to the next question. There will be time to return to the other question later. Get everything done that can be done, first, to guarantee all the grades that can be compiled, and to build all of the confidence possible. Then return to the weaker questions to build the marks from there.

Remember, one's own reality can be created, so as long as the belief is there, success will follow. And remember: anxiety can happen later, right now, there's an exam to be written!

After the examination is complete, whether there is a feeling for a good grade or a bad grade, don't dwell on the exam, and be certain to follow through on the reward that was promised...and enjoy it! Don't dwell on any mistakes that have been made, as there is nothing that can be done at this point anyway.

Additionally, don't begin to study for the next test right away. Do something relaxing for a while, and let the mind relax and prepare itself to begin absorbing information again.

From the results of the exam - both the grade and the entire experience, be certain to learn from what has gone on. Perfect studying habits and work some more on confidence in order to make the next examination experience even better than the last one.

Learn to avoid places where openings occurred for laziness, procrastination and day dreaming.

Use the time between this exam and the next one to better learn to relax, even learning to relax on cue, so that any anxiety can be controlled during the next exam. Learn how to relax the body. Slouch in your chair if that helps. Tighten and then relax all of the different muscle groups, one group at a time, beginning with the feet and then working all the way up to the neck and face. This will ultimately relax the muscles more than they were to begin with. Learn how to breathe deeply and comfortably, and focus on this breathing going in and out as a relaxing thought. With every exhale, repeat the word "relax."

As common as test anxiety is, it is very possible to overcome it. Make yourself one of the test-takers who overcome this frustrating hindrance.

Additional Bonus Material

Due to our efforts to try to keep this book to a manageable length, we've created a link that will give you access to all of your additional bonus material.

Please visit http://www.mometrix.com/bonus948/ncctncpt to access the information.